Illness in Context

At the Interface

Volume 65
A volume in the *Making Sense Of* series
'Health, Illness and Disease'

Probing the Boundaries

Illness in Context

Edited by
Knut Stene-Johansen and Frederik Tygstrup

Rodopi

Amsterdam - New York, NY 2010

The paper on which this book is printed meets the requirements of "ISO 9706:1994, Information and documentation - Paper for documents - Requirements for permanence".

ISBN: 978-90-420-2943-9
E-Book ISBN: 978-90-420-2944-6

Printed in the Netherlands

CONTENTS

Acknowledgements

Hélène Cixous, The Day I Wasn't There. Translated by Beverley Bic Brahic. Evanston: Northwestern University Press, 2006. Pp. 25-39.

Illness in Context

Knut Stene-Johansen and Frederik Tygstrup

> Illness is the night-side of life, a more onerous citizenship. Everyone who is born holds dual citizenship, in the kingdom of the well and in the kingdom of the sick. Although we all prefer to use only the good passport, sooner or later each of us is obliged, at least for a spell, to identify ourselves as citizens of that other place.
>
> Susan Sontag, *Illness as Metaphor*

This book is a contribution to humanistic studies of illness. Medical humanities are by nature cross-disciplinary, and in recent years studies in this field have been recognized as a platform for dialogue between the 'two cultures' of the natural sciences and the humanities. Contemporary cultural studies have put an increasing emphasis on the interaction of scientific insights and the cultural forms of language and historical everyday life. Likewise, it is becoming commonly acknowledged that medical research should focus on disease not only as a clinical-biological phenomenon in keeping with the modern professionalizing of medicine under the aegis of biological science, but also on its perception from a first-person perspective, through actual accounts, narratives and experiences. Contemporary medical humanities have their origin in this dialogue and promote an exchange among a wide array of disciplines, from sociology, aesthetics, history, anthropology, philosophy, cultural studies, comparative literature, feminist theory and the branches of applied medicine and medical care to the core sciences of biology, psychiatry, neurology and cognitive science.

The relationship between medicine and the humanities has changed throughout the disciplines' histories. Our opinion is that the meeting of medicine and the humanities can be mutually beneficial to the degree that they have certain principles in common. One of these shared principles can be sought in earlier medicine, in the classical Hippocratic practices based on the holistic idea of the human being, wherein symptomology appeared as a humanistic common theory of the sign. Basically, illness has two different appearances: the general *knowledge* about illness and the specific *experience* of illness. These perspectives correspond to the two cultures. The relationship between these two appearances is historical. Illness as a biological reality is embedded in historical forms of understanding and thinking that in turn condition the manner in which the biological reality can be the object of experience. The task is to bring them into dialogue, in contrast to the traditional priority given to knowledge over experience, and to focus on their shared characteristics and the historical modes of their interaction.

This book is a result of an encounter of several disciplines, including medicine, history and literature. The main stress is on the literary perspectives of the interdisciplinary collaboration. The reading practices highlighting the clinical, phenomenological and archeological approaches to illness take as their point of departure the living text, that is, the literary experience mediated and created by the text. Literature is seen not solely as a medium for the representation of experiences of illness, but also as a historical praxis involved in the forging of our common understanding of illness. In contrast to traditional literary analysis – primarily oriented toward the interpretation of the literary work's meaning – the project will emphasize description and understanding of how literature itself performs as a means of interpretation of reality.

From the bifocal perception on medicine and literature we are interested in analyzing what role literature plays in answering the question of what illness really is. What is the importance of narration and what does the formal universe of literature mean in this context? At the same time we will emphasize some of the cultural understandings attached to different historical images of illness using the methods of comparative literature. This inquiry will be elaborated in both studies of literary works and case studies, for example of hysteria understood as a cultural diagnosis, insanity as an historical notion, the ideas associated with illnesses such as tuberculosis, or cardiology's philosophical and historical underpinnings.

The phenomenon of illness is dependent on the context in which it is assessed. In this book, we have singled out three different contextual layers: the individual, the cultural and the institutional (or epistemological). The interrelations among the three are important. The individual context for experiencing illness is inscribed in a larger cultural context that also includes the institution (i.e. medicine as science and as practice) which in turn conditions the possibility of articulating any subjective experience. The essays in this book will attempt to shed light on the significance of the different contexts and their complex internal relations.

Against this background of illness as a historically contingent phenomenon, the overriding inquiry of this book is of illness in its historical mode of existence. This understanding of illness suggests a three-pronged analytical approach. The first is the analysis of knowledge, the historical epistemology at work in clinical reflection and forms of experience. The second is the ensuing analysis of power, of the historical institutions that dominate cultural expression of illness's double objectivity. The third, finally, is an analysis of different forms of self-knowledge, the modes of thematizing individual experience permitted in a given culture.

Accordingly, the book has been divided into three sections on clinic, phenomenology, and archeology. The anthology opens on the concept of the clinic as the place where a patient is received and treated, but also the place where a specific experience is articulated and discussed. In the clinic, we meet a manifest dynamic between the sign, the symptom and the interpretation, as in the discussion of problems associated with diagnosis in general and of the differences between evidence-based and narrative medicine. Thus this section will focus also on medical and health education, while laying out a framework for the interpretive activity to follow in the subsequent sections.

The section on phenomenology is devoted to literary and cultural approaches to illness through analyses of literary representations of the relationship between interpretation and diagnosis. As the term 'phenomenology' indicates, the point of departure is the idea that the world appears to us in the form of experience, which can be the object of a particular type of reflection that emphasizes the experiential aspect. Based on this understanding the essays in this section address the human life-world where illness is inscribed in a meaning-conferring context. Furthermore, the phenomenological approach implies a philosophical or theoretical understanding of existence, wherein the question of what illness is can appear to require an ontological answer. As the basis for such questions, literature will be regarded as a pivotal point of experience and reflection, embedded in the forms of language and narrative.

The section on archeology will retrieve some historical configurations of the knowledge and experience of illness and expose fragments of archives where illness and medical knowledge have been inscribed. The notion of archeology will thus broaden the historical dimension into the histories of ideas, of medicine and of literature. These examples of singular historical contexts of illness should not be seen as definitive historical tableaux, but rather as sketches of contextual frames into which literary practices intervene to create images of historical experience.

The three concepts that organize the book are lines of approach to one overarching subject. What we wish to outline is both the individual profiles of the clinical, the phenomenological and the archeological contexts and their complex internal configurations. It is important to see the three terms as related and to draw lines among the points they constitute: from the clinic to phenomenology and archeology, from phenomenology to the clinic and archeology, and from archeology to the clinic and phenomenology. With an allusion to hospital organization, we could see it as a question of three wards, but as we have also seen, of three doorways into a common room.

The essays of the book navigate between literature and medicine by considering medicine as historical knowledge and literature as a contribution to the historical production of forms of human experience. The understanding of literature as a historical production of experience includes methods of interpreting and expressing a human reality. This is partly a question of how literature voices testimony of illness experience, and partly of how literature constructs forms that allow reflection and rewrite experience in particular ways. That illness has two kinds of objectivity – clinical and phenomenological – is not to say that they are essentially different or mutually exclusive. A crucial aim of the book is indeed to show how they are connected. The perspective of such an investigation is to consider the different dimensions of subjectivity and take into account the clinical and phenomenological historical dimensions whose components correspond to the original forms of *gnosis* and *praxis*, that is, knowledge and practice. The understanding of medicine as a historical form of knowledge includes both the inner order of the discourses of medicine and natural science, and the ways in which they resonate in the cultural, artistic, juridical and political spheres surrounding them. Our aim is to demonstrate from different angles how the relationship between the two kinds of objectivities mentioned above is organized, represented and essentially mediated in literature and in a variety of literary perceptions.

The double object of our inquiry thus opens up an area of analysis that includes medical-historical and humanistic studies, wider topics in cultural studies and narrower topics in art and literary analysis. It is nonetheless crucial for us to highlight that these traditionally separate areas should be considered not only according to their specific and quite different profiles, but also as historically interrelated fields, and that precisely the inquiry into these transversal relations might shed new light on the very nature of illness.

1. The Essays

The essays collected in this volume are intended to demonstrate the different contextual layers that surround the basic phenomenon of illness. Although the essays can in no way be said to cover a salient number of cases, they nonetheless demonstrate how the construction of contextual knowledge should take into consideration the perspective outlined by the three aspects – clinical, phenomenological and archeological – and their interactions.

The first article opens the Clinic section with concrete situations and teaching practices in humanistic illness research. In her article 'The search for meaning in modern medicine', Deborah Kirklin argues that an approach to ethical analysis that combines an enhanced appreciation of the context in which illness is experienced with an acknowledgement of the highly constructed and inter-subjective nature of moral reasoning has something of value to offer to impartial ethicists. The issues are examined through the new genetics, end of life issues, organ donation, reproductive medicine and women's health. Kirklin outlines a practical approach, drawing on theory and grounded in clinical practice, and she argues that enhancing appreciation of the context of ethical issues – by informing the ethicist's choice of framing, language and narrative constructs – has the potential to alter the nature of the ethical debate.

Jan Frich's article 'Dialogue and creativity: narrative in the clinical encounter', discusses recent developments in 'narrative-based medicine', arguing that that the concept of 'healing dramas' captures essential aspects of the clinical encounter, and supplements the approach in which the patient is conceptualized as 'text'. The healing drama offers conceptual tools that help us to understand processes in which narratives are performed in clinical settings. This approach reveals the active role physicians also have as producers and co-authors of 'text' in clinical encounters. Frich's text is centered on a narrative constructed on the basis of the his own clinical experience as a neurosurgeon. The article highlight the hermeneutic character of diagnostic reasoning in clinical medicine, and particularly discusses the tension between 'cases' and 'dramas'.

In her 'Clinical tales and the art-like creativity of the body' Drude von der Fehr explores the possibility that a person can live in an 'aesthetic' world. She bases her exploration on two clinical autobiographies of the Russian neuropsychologist A. R. Luria. The question of whether there is an art-like life-world approaches a possible connection between aesthetic immediacy and the development of the brain. Von der Fehr argues that to live a style or to live in the world of art might be painful, and might represent a loss of biological capacity. On the other hand, the study of such states might open up for new hypothesizes in medical reasoning.

In 'Signs of illness/pathologies of interpretation' Vincent Colapietro states that illness is, first and foremost, a modification of our orientation toward the everyday, and that the relevant phenomena – the most salient ways in which illness reveals itself – are in effect somatic signs, broadly conceived. The investigation of illness in this and indeed any other legitimate sense depends, above all else, on the complex interplay between two dynamic factors: the free play of the theoretical imagination and a fidelity to disclosures of experience. Colapietro claims that the medical and literary discourses can contribute to both of these factors. The most pathological frameworks of interpretation, he says, are precisely those that occlude the *fateful paradoxes of illness* in their irreducibly paradoxical and uniquely fateful character. Literature is especially effective in making these occlusions visible, exposing this pathology of interpretation.

As the first text in the Phenomenology section, an excerpt from Hélène Cixous' memoir-novel *The Day I Wasn't There* describes an incident that gives us an idea of how complex the individual experience with illness can be. The narrator, who resembles Cixous herself, reflects upon the premature death of her first-born child, a Down's syndrome baby. The story takes place in Algeria, and Cixous lets the narrator use this event to explore her own family history: her mother is a refugee from Nazi Germany, her brother a student at medical school, the baby takes its name from her dead grandfather. Cixous thus, in her poetic, provocative and beautiful style manages to pose some crucial questions about our relationships to illness, death, family history and women's inner landscapes.

In 'Henri Michaux's great health' Gérard Danou reflects upon Michaux's statement that he painted and wrote 'for his good health'. Yet, due to his weak heart, Michaux suffered ill-health all his life. However, not heeding medical advice, he did not spare himself for over 80 years. As he put it, his only drug was 'feeling tired'! By means of 'pen strokes', Michaux lay on paper the innumerable aspects of his psycho-somatic suffering, thereby both exorcizing and alchemizing it through the poetic act. His work focuses on the narcissistic self and phenomenological body awareness: 'Cœnesthésie, mare nostrum', as Michaux says. But this did not prevent him from having an accurate perception of other people and of the world, at a distance. By an alchemical process, he appropriated and operated a value-transmutation of the scientific and medical languages of the twentieth century for his personal use. He thus offers an unclassifiable and open-ended poetry, resistant to all abuses of single interpretations, especially those of the medical world. According to his poetry function, the 'non-breathable becomes breathable and the unlivable becomes livable'. Michaux's whole output is an exercise in perfection, Danou writes, a medicine for oneself, a Nietzschean healing pedagogy, that is to say 'good health'.

In 'American dementia, dying in a blue chair', Frederik Tygstrup introduces that the blue chair where the father of the protagonist siblings in Jonathan Franzen's novel *The Corrections* ends his life. It is a comfortable, restful and utterly ugly chair – the only piece of furniture of his own acquisition in an American suburban home – and the last confine of a misspent existence that has lost its directions through forced retirement and soon flees into precocious dementia. From having been a marginal and rather inconspicuous disease, dementia, especially in the guise of Alzheimer's disease, has become one of the major challenges to health-care in the industrialized world during the last 20 or so years. Tygstrup's article examines some of the ways in which the rapidly increasing number of patients with the diagnosis of dementia is reflected in contemporary American fiction. Through a reading of three novels – *The Corrections*, Amy Tan's *The Bonesetters Daughter* and Chuck Palahniuk's *Choke* – Tygstrup discusses how dementia highlights some more general features in contemporary culture, especially the changing role of cultural memory in a uniform consumer culture, the blurring boundaries between the real and the imaginary in a media-saturated society and the transformation of generational authority in a youth-idealizing culture. Tygstrup argues that the role of literature in relation to dementia can be seen not only as a phenomenological first-person approach to the experience of patients and relatives, but also as a diagnosis of some cultural predicaments underlying the spread of the clinical syndrome, and not least some strategies for coping with the disease in this expanded cultural context.

In 'Tolstoy and the making of the inhuman', Knut Stene-Johansen claims that texts about illness and death may show how something unreasonable in a given literary text may have its own, profound reason. Both a slow, progressive demise brought on by illness and a sudden death us something about how an ending can manifest itself long before the final, full stop is set. This oscillation between life and death – where the unreasonable, accidental and causally unclear in the symptom's appearance become the only reason for the text – is well illustrated in Leo Tolstoy's novella 'The Death of Ivan Ilyich'. When the actual illness is impossible to define as more than just an illness, says Stene-Johansen, a specific problem arises concerning the very role of illness in human existence, of which 'Ivan Ilich' is an example. The novella's subject is the 'material', inauthentic life of the bourgeoisie, but it also deals with illness as a starting point for a change in the way of living, breaking from the idea of death as only the death of 'Man' in a Heideggerian sense.

Anne Kveim Lie opens the Archeology section with 'Constructing the Norwegian Radesyge: experience, politics and practice in the radesyge hospitals'. The 'radesyge' was a disease of considerable importance in Norwegian medical history. The disease resulted in the opening of the first hospitals in Norway with a therapeutic intention, and was also the first subject to be treated in scholarly works in Norway. In its historiography, *radesyge* was assumed to be a kind of tertiary syphilis. In her article, Anne Helene Kveim Lie discuss the rise of the radesyge hospitals in the 1770s. The history of these hospitals has never been written, although in all reference works their constitution in passing is emphasized as one of the key events in Norwegian medical history. In this traditional account the radesyge hospitals are highlighted as important elements in the scientific development, and as steps towards a more rational health care system in Norway. But what is this 'scientific development'? And how, if it is so, did the hospitals contribute to this development? What was taking place inside these walls that implied a change in hospital function? These are some of the questions Anne Helene Kveim Lie discusses.

In 'Metaphors, figures and description in Sénac's *Traité de la structure du cœur, de son action et de ses maladies* (1749)', Eric Hamraouï writes that in his famous treatise Jean-Bertrand Sénac (1693-1770), Louis XV's first physician, gives equal importance to the manifestation of the meaning via discourse and representation. 'The expression of the image is just as decisive as the expression of the language', Sénac says. Hamraouï discusses how Sénac contradicts the thesis of the native inferiority of the image – a pale reflection or imperfect mimesis of the reality it pictures – compared to the text. He also claims that Sénac shows the impossibility of dissociating the analysis of the discursive forms and the metaphors that strengthen their persuasive power from the study of meaning provided by anatomical representation the gaps between it and the discourse that introduces or comments on it. But then, how can one define the modes of articulation of the two majors forms of mediation of knowledge and practice that are language and image in Sénac's treatise?

In 'Who's afraid of Amalie Skram? Hysteria and rebellion in Amalie Skram's novels of mental hospitals', Hilde Bondevik sheds light on hysteria as a cultural diagnosis by examining two 1895 novels set in mental hospitals: *Professor Hieronimus* and *På St. Jørgen,* by the Norwegian-Danish author Amalie Skram. Bonevik's discussion deploys an understanding of hysteria as a typical illness and diagnosis of the time and as a form of hysterization of female disorder and rebellion. Amalie Skram's own experience constitutes a framework for the article, suggesting that Skram may be regarded as an important figure in intellectual history, embodying the spirit of her age and helping to draft a new and modern female typology.

In 'A wave rushing from the South; The great influenza in Jacob Paludan's *Jørgen Stein*' Mette Kia Krabbe Meyer notes that in 1918 the world faced a challenge as the 'Spanish flu' swept the shores and lands of all countries. Scientists struggled to define the disease and citizens experienced a change in interpersonal relationships due to the fear of infection while they at the same time lived through sickness and death of dear ones. The Danish writer Jacob Paludan included the influenza in his novel *Jørgen Stein*, which when published in 1932 was heralded as a factual description of provincial Denmark at the time of World War I. As one reads the book today, however, it becomes clear that its realism is a sticky affair. As for the influenza, the doubts, grief and ethical dilemmas of the epidemic largely give way to a definition of infection along the lines of the moral and sexual taboos established in the description of syphilis in cultural and literary history, for instance in the works of Thomas Mann. Paludan thus offers an account which is more or less a story of dubious culprits and crime scenes. Meyer's argument is that if the novel is to be regarded as a factual description of the influenza and its psychological consequences, it is as much due to its manifestation of a certain cultural reaction to the influenza, as to any detailed description of the epidemic.

In 'Pathogenesis: life, literature, animality; medical theory and biological nihilism in eighteenth-century thought' by Johan Redin, we learn that there is an attraction to the idea of the post-human in the history and theory of vitalism. Throughout the eighteenth and nineteenth centuries there was a lively discussion about not only the origin and nature of humankind, but also of its future and progress. The belief in biological teleology was seriously challenged by the temptations of biological nihilism. The debate, which initially concerned mostly materialists, opened up for radically new ideas of the concept of life and the evolution of humans. Turning to Friedrich Schiller, Karl Philipp Moritz and Honoré de Balzac, Redin's essay explores the role of medical theory in the history of aesthetics and the traces of biological nihilism in literature and philosophy.

2. Target Group

The target group for this book comprises professional in the various disciplines, and students of health and culture. It has been our aim that the book contribute to teaching in humanistic illness research, and function as a topical resource book that formulates controversial problems in the crucial meeting of medicine and the humanities.

I - CLINIC

The Search for Meaning in Modern Medicine

Deborah Kirklin

Abstract
This chapter will argue that an approach to ethical analysis which combines an enhanced appreciation of the context within which illness is experienced with an acknowledgement of the highly constructed and inter-subjective nature of moral reasoning has something of value to offer to impartialist ethicists. Examples will be given of how this approach can be used in practice, both when using reason to address ethical problems or issues that arise in medicine or the life sciences and when exploring these concerns in educational settings. The following areas of modern medicine will be used to examine these issues: the new genetics, end of life issues, organ donation, reproductive medicine, and women's health. Examples will be given of educational initiatives that use the arts and humanities to provide a human context for medicine and for the moral decisions that its practice involves. The examples given are chosen in an attempt to illustrate the need to ask searching questions about context, framing, and meaning, if the application of impartialist ethical principles is to lead to both sound and persuasive analyses. A practical approach will be outlined which draws on these theoretical ideas and is grounded in clinical practice. It will be argued that an enhanced appreciation of the context for ethical issues, by informing the ethicist's choice of framing, language and narrative construct, has the potential to alter the nature of the ethical debate. Moreover, it will be argued that this approach can enable a cogent analysis of the immanence of power relations within health care, and that understanding these power relations is an essential step in determining what matters to those affected by illness, and to ensuring that their voice is heard.

Key Words: Context; ethical analysis; framing; life science; meaning; medicine; power relations.

*****

1. Introduction

If you are interested in and enjoy thinking about the ethical problems that arise in medicine or the life sciences then this chapter has been written for you. Whether you are from a philosophical, medical or lay background I hope to encourage you to turn a literary eye on the ethical arguments you hear or make in the future. Throughout this chapter I will use the term medical ethicist to refer to anyone using reason to address these ethical issues.

The approach I will describe, whilst grounded in clinical practice, draws on insights and methodologies from literary studies. This approach, which will be familiar to medical humanities scholars and educators, is based on the assumption that an ethical analysis informed by a wider understanding of the context within which illness and health care are experienced and delivered will be a richer and more nuanced one. I will argue that an enhanced appreciation of the context for these ethical issues, by informing the ethicist's choice of framing, language and narrative construct, has the potential to alter the nature of the ethical debate. Moreover I will argue that this approach to ethical analysis can enable a cogent analysis of power relations within health care. Understanding these power relations is an essential step in determining what matters to those affected by illness, and to ensuring that their voice is heard.

2. The Search for Meaning

The attempt to understand both the purpose and goals of medicine and, importantly, how these relate to and affect both individuals and societies, is at the heart of medical ethical inquiry. This search for meaning can be aided by an examination of the language employed when clinical practice and the ethical issues it poses are discussed. In addition to examining the words that are spoken, an examination of the words that are not spoken, and the reasons why they are not, can also be rewarding. Michel Foucault addressed the relationship between the words and ideas contained in a narrative, and those excluded in the editing and selecting involved in the process of producing a narrative, in volume one of his treatise on the history of sexuality when he said,

> There is no binary division to be made between what one says and what one does not say; we must try to determine the different ways of not saying such things, how those who can and those who cannot speak them are distributed, which type of discourse is authorised, or which form of discretion is required in either case. There is not one but many silences, and they are an integral part of the strategies that underlie and permeate discourses.[1]

Clearly any discussion of unspoken words is necessarily speculative, but if Foucault is correct, then the task of the reader is to try and understand what is not said as well as what is said, and to try and understand who is empowered to speak and who is not. To do this requires the reader to recognise that all narratives are a way of not saying things. I hope to show that this approach may offer useful insights into the functioning, or indeed malfunctioning, of the doctor-patient dynamic and health care delivery. I will suggest that some words may be unacceptable, unbearable, or unspeakable. I have examined the origins of the painful and uncomfortable nature of these words, and the implications of this discomfort, at length, elsewhere.[2 3 4]

It is important to make clear that although this chapter include many examples from clinical practice it remains, nevertheless, a chapter about medical ethics and not about clinical practice. When I talk of wanting the patient's voice to be heard I am not advocating a system of clinical care that places all patients on the psychiatric couch, whether they want to be there or not, and extracts from them their innermost feelings and thoughts. Instead I am arguing that ethical arguments constructed with an informed appreciation of the context within which illness is experienced and health care delivered are more likely to reflect what matters to the interested parties. It is in this sense that I will argue that the patient's voice needs to be heard.

Far from intending to alienate clinical readers by making this distinction I am instead assuming that many if not all of them will be captured by my definition of a medical ethicist. Furthermore, whilst the argument I am making is philosophical in nature I believe it has practical implications for both individual practitioners and for the way in which health care is organised. For this reason I believe that an interdisciplinary dialogue between the humanities and medicine has potential benefits for us all.

3. Foucault and the Use of Parentheses

> (The) patient is only an external fact; the medical reading must take him into account only to place him in parentheses.
>
> Michel Foucault [5]

Michel Foucault's metaphor, in which patients are placed in parentheses, expresses his analysis of one of the ways in which doctors try to recognise and characterise patterns of illness and behaviour, despite the confusing individuality of how people respond to and express ill health. In an attempt to be objective, doctors risk removing from the equation the individual factors that underlie the very different ways in which people respond to ill health.

In an attempt to be rational and objective, and, possibly, in order to avoid the charge of moral relativism, ethicists also seek to categorise and characterise ethical dilemmas. This approach is intended to minimise the impact of the confusing individuality of the context within which ethically challenging problems exist: the backdrop for the real and practical problems faced by actual human individuals living rich and complicated lives. Foucault's metaphor can be extended, by analogy, to argue that the patient, doctor, and other interested parties, can all too often be placed in parentheses by ethicists whose arguments place little value on the individual context within which patients exist, doctors practice, and society makes decisions about advances in biotechnology, or health care delivery.

As in medicine, this bracketing by the ethicist may of course serve a valuable role in allowing general arguments to be developed, and patterns to be recognised. But if these general arguments cannot be generally applied, because they fail to take account of matters of great importance to the individuals they are meant to guide, then an impasse may be swiftly reached. Useful as the devise of bracketing can be, as Foucault makes clear, something important is lost in the process. In the case of doctors this something is the person whose trust they must gain if advice is to be heeded and treatment complied with. For the ethicist this something is the person whom they wish to convince of the validity of their arguments. Despite the logic employed the conclusions are simply, for that individual, counterintuitive and therefore unacceptable.

4. The Gap between Logic and Intuition

This gap between logic and intuition is perhaps most easily exemplified by the debate between those who consider abortion morally permissible (often characterised and labelled as pro-choice) and those who consider abortion morally impermissible (often characterised and labelled as pro-life). Each of these terms pro-choice and pro-life are implicitly positive labels declaring what the proponents are in favour of rather than what they might wish to prohibit. Indeed it is difficult to imagine that those on either side of this debate would wish to declare themselves respectively against either choice or life. The use of these labels frames this debate by reinforcing the already polarised stances of each side and invites opponents to condemn themselves by challenging either the concept of choice, equivalent in this case to the right to self determination, or the idea that life is something of value. Rather than pursuing the argument either for or against these two opposing viewpoints, what I am here interested in is the consequences of re-framing these labels.

One, linguistically logical, counterpart to the term pro-choice is anti-choice, and to pro-life anti-life with both of these alternative framings implicit in the more accepted framing of pro-choice and pro-life. The consequences of the premises and values that lead to the current framing pro-choice versus pro-life – are an inevitable gap between logic and intuition. Those who argue against abortion (pro-life) usually begin from the premise that all human life, from conception, is intrinsically valuable and ought not to be destroyed. For them a life begins with conception and the value they place on this human life is greater than the value they place on autonomy, in this case that of the pregnant woman. They are not anti-choice so much as anti the choice to end human life. Those who are pro-choice value personhood rather than humanness per se. For them a person is a self-conscious being, aware of itself as existing over time and place. They therefore value life but consider the life of an embryo, for them devoid of personhood, to be of less value than the autonomy of a pregnant woman. Both those who are pro-choice and those who are pro-life appear to begin from the same premises: that the lives of people are of value and that it is good to respect the autonomy of people. But this apparent agreement over the starting premises is illusory because the two sides mean something very different by the word person. One way to understand the impasse that these opposing parties find themselves in is to examine the linguistic consequences of using biological discourse to make normative arguments: put simply, since the two sides are talking different languages it should be no surprise if they don't understand each other.[6] This same impasse is rehearsed equally well in the debate over euthanasia.

Another type of gap between logic and intuition can occur when doctors or other health care professionals are expected to request permission for the use of the organs of a brain stem dead patient for transplantation into other patients unknown, either personally or professionally, to that doctor. Logically, the doctor in question may well see organ transplantation as something of value and wish to enable those in need of organs to receive them. However research evidence shows that some doctors find themselves emotionally ill equipped to make these requests. I have suggested elsewhere that the origins of the dis-ease that some doctors feel about asking grieving relatives for permission to remove and use the organs of a person who until then the doctor had been responsible for caring for are culturally embedded and that asking invokes ancient taboos.[5] I likened the process of asking relatives for permission to use organs to the breaking of taboos that anatomical dissection involves and argued that if we want doctors to ask relatives for permission to use organs for transplantation then we should first acknowledge that these taboos exist and then explain why we still want them broken. Failure to do so will lead some people to avoid asking even if, logically, they know why they should.

The types of gap between logic and intuition that I am here concerned with therefore include not only gaps between what two opposing sides argue in a given case, such as abortion, but also the gaps that are exposed by the differences between what people are told by the prevailing moral codes, either within medicine or within society, that they ought to do and what they in fact choose to do or express a desire to do.

5. Bridging the Gap

Who or what must the ethicist understand in order to try and bridge the gap between logic and intuition? What is it about a person that the ethicist needs to understand, and to connect with, in order to achieve a shared understanding on which progress can be made? One answer to this question is offered by, amongst others, Alasdair MacIntyre. MacIntyre argues that individuals seek narrative order within their lives.[7] He defines this as a human need for individuals to feel that the events in their lives, and the role they play, are consistent with the values they hold, the emotional commitments they have to others, and the wider historical context or order of things. MacIntyre argues that this need for narrative coherence is an essential component of the search for meaning in life so characteristic of human beings. If MacIntyre is right then, in theory at least, a logical argument which makes sense within the narrative construct for the individual patient or doctor is more likely to make sense to that individual, to convince not just on an intellectual level but also on an intuitive one.

This line of argument is not of course unique to MacIntyre, or indeed to those philosophers traditionally associated with narrative approaches to medical ethics. Bernard Williams, for example, argued that success in creating and delivering a system of morality that is truly impartial would come at a high price, with many of the factors people consider most important in their lives excluded from consideration.[8] Williams argued that these excluded factors are the very things that often inspire individuals to take moral goals seriously. Whilst an impartial analysis of ethical concerns may require the removal or placing in parentheses of these individual factors, convincing on an intuitive level of the validity of the conclusions so carefully reached would appear to require these individual factors to be added back in.[9]

In relation to women's health, for example, an impartial application of the principle of equity to the delivery of health care to female patients, devoid of a detailed analysis of the context within which female patients access health care, male and female doctors deliver that care, and medical research is undertaken, risks becoming an empty if fine ideal of little help to either patients or doctors.[10] Ignoring this context can lead to the misleading conclusion that any inequities in health care provision, relative to gender, can be remedied simply by ensuring that health care practitioners treat both men and women without favour or prejudice. This laudable goal is unachievable unless the historical, cultural, political, and psychological context of what I have call the sexual demographics of health[18] are recognised and acknowledged.

6. Laying Bare Human Frailties

It is also important to recognise the emotional and psychological baggage that doctors and other health care professionals bring with them to their encounter with the patient, and to explore the influence these personal factors have on how professional careers interact with patients, and perceive and respond to moral dilemmas. Rather than trying to place this non-professional part of the doctor in parentheses, I have argued elsewhere that recognising this baggage, for example the doctor's concerns and fears regarding her own mortality, is of fundamental importance if moral imperatives such as 'tell the truth' are to be complied with.[3] Not only can it be harder for a doctor to impart painful facts if she has not addressed or recognised her own concerns but her understanding of what constitutes 'the truth' may be affected by this lack of self awareness. Virtue ethics[11], whilst recognising the key role of the individual in applying moral principles, can appear to have little tolerance for the imperfections of those individuals. In laying bare some of these human frailties I am not calling for an ever more rigorous attempt to suppress them, but instead for an acknowledgment, by patients, doctors, and ethicists, that these weaknesses are at the same time often the source of strength and motivation in acts of goodness and kindness.

7. Framing: Why it Matters

Economists, psychologists and literature scholars, attribute great importance to framing. They argue that framing matters a great deal and challenge the idea that the decisions individuals make, about the equivalence or otherwise of alternate choices, are objective. Psychologists Daniel Kahneman and Amos Tversky have shown experimentally that the way in which factually identical information is presented to individuals can have surprising consequences for the choices they make.[12] [13] One example involved research participants being asked to consider the merits of implementing a new immunisation programme, and whether they would wish it to be introduced as a public health measure. By re-framing the same facts – in the first case by focussing on the lives that would be saved if the programme were implemented, and in the second by focussing on the lives that would not be saved even if the programme were implemented- the researchers were able to make two identical propositions appear unequal in their appeal. When the question was framed such that the lives lost were emphasised, respondents did not favour the new programme. When the question was framed such that the lives saved were emphasised respondents did favour the proposed programme.

Economist David Kreps[14] has suggested that, per Tversky and Kahneman, this occurs because individuals tend to think of decisions as deviations from the status quo, and that the way in which dilemmas or choices are framed establishes in the mind of the person what exactly that status quo is. In the first framing it was established in respondents' minds that without the programme 600 people would die and the status quo was thereby established of 600 dead. Given this status quo the saving of 200 lives by the implementation of the immunisation programme is seen as an improvement. In the second framing the status quo is established as being before these predicted deaths, so that prior to the immunisation programme no one is dead. Even though the immunisation programme will save 200 lives, by the end of the programme 400 others will have died. This deviation from the status quo is not perceived as an improvement.

If this re-framing can have such profound implications for the choices people make, then concerns about the influence of framing on ethical decision making would seem reasonable. Indeed John Nash's game theory,[15] which concerns the influence that framing has on the choices individuals make, has been of great theoretical interest not only to economists[16] but also to philosophers, with the prisoner's dilemma being the most famous example of this.[17] It could of course be argued that given long enough to think about the two framings of the immunisation scenario outlined above that there would be less apparent inconsistency in the answers given. If however a particular individual were to reconsider their response, this change of mind, either to proceed with or prohibit the proposed immunisation programme, would, I suggest, be preceded by a reframing of the proposition. Thus the 'save 200 lives' would need to be reframed as '400 die' in order to lose appeal, and the '400 die' would likewise need reframing as 'save 200 lives' to become appealing.

i. Reframing and the MMR Vaccine

A contemporary example of the way in which framing can influence the choices people make concerns the on-going controversy surrounding the triple vaccine for measles, mumps and rubella: the MMR vaccine. I have no wish to examine the scientific merits or otherwise of the research into the possible links between the vaccine and autism, suffice it to say, for the sake of this discussion, that significant numbers of members of the public believe that in rare but tragic cases a child will develop autism following administration of the MMR vaccine.

In common with most general practitioners a number of these families are patients of mine and in all the cases I am familiar with these parents in no sense belittle the serious and sometimes fatal consequences of infection with the measles virus. Whilst many parents have found ways to access single vaccines, many have not and have instead left their children unvaccinated. For these parents, whose children remain unvaccinated, the possibility that their child might suffer from autism amounts to a deviation from the status quo (well child) and they therefore reject vaccination.

Although the evidence that MMR is a causal agent in autism is unconvincing what is really interesting here is the effect of framing on how the issue is perceived by some parents. Immunisation, in general, is after all not without acknowledged risk. All immunisation programmes carry some morbidity and mortality. That this is understood by at least some parents is evidenced by the many questions parents ask about side effects, and the implications of, for example, egg allergies or swellings at previous vaccination sites. What seems to have occurred in the MMR debate is a reframing of the dilemma faced by any parent asked for consent for their child to be vaccinated. The traditional, public health, framing of immunisation is one where the high risk of something mild to very bad happening (the illness, disability and death associated with measles, mumps and rubella) is traded for the much lower risk of something mild to severe (the mild to severe side effects including death associated with all immunisation programmes). For communities with living memory or day to day experience of the ravages of diseases, such as polio, measles, and tuberculosis, the risks that immunisation seeks to minimise are the status quo and, as evidenced by the WHO immunisation programmes in developing countries, when vaccination programmes are available uptake is high. Nowadays, in developed countries, there is, at least amongst the current generation of young parents, little memory of these diseases but a raised awareness of autism. It is perhaps for some of these parents easier to imagine autism afflicting their child than it is to imagine measles once more becoming a killer disease.

ii. Framing Ethical Arguments

An objective examination of the way in which arguments are framed can be revealing about the value systems and assumptions of those doing the framing. Consciously or subconsciously, individuals frame their arguments to achieve specific and desired effects. The choices individuals make about how to frame arguments are, I believe, a natural and logical consequence of the beliefs and values held by those individuals. Public health officials advocating the implementation of a new immunisation programme are likely to emphasis the lives that will be saved that would otherwise have been lost. General practitioners concerned at the consequences of a potential outbreak of measles, and unimpressed by the research connecting MMR and autism, are likely to emphasise the protection immunisation offers against a potentially deadly disease.

It is, of course, possible for an argument to be framed in a way that seeks to mislead others about the value systems and assumptions of the person proposing the argument, again with specific and desired effects in mind. Here the term spin is often used instead of frame with the term spin implying that a degree of duplicity and manipulation is involved. Although spin is a fascinating subject I will avoid the use of this rather pejorative term. For the sake of this chapter I am interested in the role that framing plays in the honest and sincere attempts of ethicists to make soundly reasoned and persuasive arguments.

A detailed example of the intellectual gains that consideration of framing can have for ethicists, showing how the choice of language used to initiate an important consultation exercise about cloning not only revealed the underlying pro-attitudes of the authors but could also be used to predict the conclusions subsequently reached, is available elsewhere.[4]

8. The Patient as Text

An important idea that merits discussion in this chapter is the suggestion that the patient is a text that the doctor must read. This metaphor, like all metaphors, requires an act of imagination, albeit one familiar to literary scholars. Again, this analysis does not need to imply that patients should be required to submit to some sort of psychological analysis by doctors. Instead, what I am here concerned with is the questions that unpacking this metaphor lead us to ask in terms of authorship of the text. This idea has been examined in detail by Kathryn Montgomery Hunter.[18]

In unpacking this metaphor it is important to remember that an ill person only becomes a patient when they seek medical care. Indeed English Law recognises a person as a patient only once a doctor has accepted responsibility for his or her care. The metaphor of the patient as text could be understood as implying that the text is embodied in the patient. In a very real sense of course the disease process does take place in the patient's body. In order to find out what form this process takes the doctor will ideally have access to what the patient has to say about how she is feeling and what has happened to her, and access to the patient's body in order to carry out physical examinations and to do further investigations. As a result of this diagnostic process the doctor will then determine what she considers the best course of action for the patient to pursue or submit to. Hunter[26] describes the text of the patient as being a constantly evolving composite: the embodied sensations and emotions the patient experiences, the story she tells to communicate these to the doctor, the retelling of the story by the doctor and other health care professionals, including the written and oral accounts given of the patient's case, the investigations undertaken, and the treatments prescribed are all inter-related parts of that text. The text of the patient is for Hunter very much a co-authored one, and the authoring of the text is the result of an inter-subjective and on-going sharing of narratives whereby each of the authors endeavours to find meaning in the narrative constructed by the other.

Howard Brody uses a slightly different but related metaphor when he suggests that the clinical encounter can be characterised as a request for help with the patient asking the doctor to help her to fix her broken story.[19] In order to work out how to help the patient to fix her broken story the doctor must first become familiar with or read the text. Note that Brody talks of helping the patient to fix her story rather than fixing it for her. This is an important point that acknowledges the value people place on being able to construct for them selves a meaningful reality from the lived experience of illness.

9. The Role of Metaphor

Ethical discourse and the language used to describe the culture and practice of medicine is of course rich with metaphor. The metaphor of patient as text is just one example. Reflection on and engagement with these metaphors can provide an opportunity to examine the tensions inherent in the doctor's role, can facilitate a clearer understanding about what medicine is and, perhaps more importantly, what it could and should be.[20] It can suggest ways of understanding what may be happening when the views and decisions of patients, families and practitioners diverge in a painful and damaging way.[21] It can raise important questions about truth telling, autonomy, and paternalism, and can challenge existing ideas about what constitutes a virtuous doctor. These ideas have attracted the attention of scholars in many academic fields including cognitive psychology, linguistics, anthropology, philosophy, literature, and history.

10. Narrative Construction and Ethical Discourse

The idea that an understanding of the structure of narrative might be important for clinicians has been explored by a number of scholars.[22] Analysing the way in which illness narratives are constructed, and by whom, can help explain why health care providers, and society in general, are often perceived, by patients and families, as paying inadequate attention to the context, or environment, within which those individuals exist. Anthropological and sociological examination of the different ways in which illness narratives can be thought about, conceptualised, or described, have led clinicians to re-evaluate the way in which they interact with patients. Applying these ideas to the work of ethicists may help them to understand why their attempts to convince on an intuitive level sometimes fail, despite the logical rigour of their reasoning. A brief overview of some of these ideas, and their potential value to ethicists, will be given next.

11. First-person Narratives of Illness

Arthur Frank, a sociologist, who has personal experience of serious illness, provides an interesting way of thinking about the interrelationship between the narrative of illness constructed by health care providers, and the first-person narrative of illness people tell about their own experiences.[23] Frank suggests that illness narratives can be thought of as having a number of different internal structures, and that understanding the nature of this structure can be useful in a number of ways.

Firstly, a comparison of the dominant narrative structure in medical illness narratives, that is those told by health care providers, and first-person illness narratives, that is those told by people who are ill, provides an indication of the priorities of each of these story-tellers. Secondly, an understanding of the internal structure of illness narratives can make it possible for those telling the stories to change the narrative construct they choose, if they so wish. Frank argues that one consequence of a failure of health care providers to recognise the important differences between the illness narrative they construct, and the illness narratives patients construct, is that people who are ill seek alternative ways of dealing with the problems posed by illness. This may, for example, involve non-compliance with treatment recommendations or the seeking of alternative care elsewhere.

Similarly, I would argue, ethicists who understand the internal structure of the narratives told by people faced with ethical conundrums, and the likewise constructed nature of the narrative that ethicists tell about these issues, are better equipped to appreciate what matters to these various interested parties. Whether this leads them to change the narrative construct they use is a different matter. A valid question would be whether what matters to the interested parties differs from what matters objectively, but begs the further question, matters to whom. My primary concern is with all those affected by illness. In the next section I provide two examples to show why generalisations about what objectively matters to individuals who are affected by illness should be made with extreme caution.

An outline of Frank's ideas about the internal structure of illness narratives follows.

12. Restitution, Chaos, and Quest Narratives

Frank suggests that one way to think about or understand illness narratives is by trying to identify what he calls the different narrative voices through which the narrative is told. He makes a number of important claims about the nature of these voices.

The voices are culturally constructed such that those wishing to tell or to enact stories have available to them a variety of ways of telling them or voices to tell them through depending on their cultural background.

These off-the-peg voices are different in different cultures. They are specific to but not exclusive to different cultures at different times.

The three narrative voices he describes are specific to contemporary North America that is to Canada and the USA.[24]

There are structural differences between the three voices of restitution, chaos, and quest narratives.

i. The Voice of the Restitution Narrative

The restitution narrative is the superficial story plot that all medical encounters could, simplistically, be summarised as:

Person is unwell

Goes to doctor/ pharmacist/ physiotherapist / acupuncturist

Seeks response that will lead to restoration of previous state of symptom free health and former social role

Arthur Frank argues that the voice of the restitution narrative casts the patient in a passive role with the health care provider as the main protagonist. He sees this as an important reason behind the fact that the voice of the restitution narrative is not dominant in first person illness narratives. He contrasts this with the dominance of the voice of the restitution narrative in the medical account of the patient's encounter with health service providers, often told through the clinical records.

ii. The Voice of the Chaos Narrative

Sometimes, indeed often, when patients are faced with serious illnesses, there is no straightforward sequence of events to re-present through a narrative, but instead only confusion and fear: here the voice of the chaos narrative is the one that dominates. According to Frank, the paradox of the voice of the chaos narrative is that it seems to be incapable of storytelling and so examples, he says, are hard to find. When considering this voice I find it helpful to think about the words that are, for all those affected by serious illness, unspeakable and unbearable. A contemplation of unspeakable and unbearable words necessarily requires an act of imagination, but can also be supported by an examination of the words that are used in illness narratives, both of patients and of professional carers. Leo Tolstoy's *The Death of Ilyich* provides a good example of a voice of chaos. Ivan Ilyich's moral agony lies in what Arthur Frank terms 'this heart of darkness' where 'the horror' cannot be told. Ivan Ilyich is a man dying of (presumably) cancer. He is in physical agony but far worse he suffers moral agony as he reaches the conclusion that he has wasted his life.

The physical, moral and spiritual agony of Ivan Ilyich stands in sharp contrast to Cicely Saunders' vision of the care that should be provided to those who are dying.[25] Cicely Saunders' vision is one in which physicians do everything in their power to minimise all of these agonies. According to her teaching, a failure to fully address these agonies is a failure of palliative care. Problematically, inherent in this philosophy is the presumption that with proper palliative care no one would choose either to end their own life or request help in doing so. Within this paradigm, a patient's desire to end her own life is interpreted not as an autonomous decision but as evidence of the failure of the palliative care team. The patient's authentic narrative is displaced by the medical narrative of palliative care with the patient no longer in control of their own circumstances but instead reliant on health professionals to 'get it right'. The irony is that by placing so much emphasis on the duty of care of health care professionals to address the needs of patients, the patient's right to autonomy is subsumed.

As Ivan Ilyich's case illustrates, not all of the causes of the agonies suffered by patients, particularly the moral and spiritual ones, will be either apparent or amenable to physician directed intervention. In these situations it is hardly surprising that patients, families, and professional carers, armed only with unbearable and unspeakable words, find themselves incapable of telling the story of the chaos they are experiencing. When I talk of patients 'telling' their story I am not, specifically, alluding to the clinical encounter, nor am I suggesting that patients be encouraged to share any more of their innermost thoughts with health care professionals then they wish to. Instead I am concerned with the power relations within medicine and society, and with those whom Foucault refers to as 'those who can and those who cannot speak'. [2]

iii. The Voice of the Quest Narrative

According to Frank, the dominant voice in most first person illness narratives is the quest narrative. For illness narratives to become sustained storytelling the voice of the quest narrative usually dominates although other voices are often mixed in.

There are three basic stages in any quest narrative

The call – when the patient recognises that a symptom is not just an indication of a disease process but is the beginning of a journey. Accepting the call means accepting that the illness will affect one's life. If the illness brings about changes this narrative is clearly not one of restitution in which the narrative is constructed in such a way that nothing, by definition, at the end of the story, will have changed.

The road of trials – the changes to one's life occur as a result of the trials that occur along this journey, including the sufferings of surgery, treatment, and the stigma and isolation that often surround illness. Trials are understood as something through which the person learns and grows and thereby these trials acquire meaning. It echoes Nietzsche's idea that: 'That which does not kill us makes us stronger.'

The return – This acquiring of meaning represents the third stage of the quest narrative, the return. Those who have experienced severe illness, such as cancer, often claim that their priorities have changed and they have greater understanding and insight about what matters in life. To quote Frank 'the self has been changed.'

iv. Being Heard

Cure and the restoration of normal physical and social function are of course of great importance to people who are ill, and so restitution is always one voice in these narratives. It is not, however, the only voice. When restoration to the person's former physical state and social role is achieved then this may well be the dominant voice and it may well be that the patient is very active in asking to be restored to this previous status quo. In these circumstances, being the passive recipient of health care may be exactly what patients actively demand. Unfortunately, serious and chronic illnesses rarely leave those experiencing them untouched, physically, psychologically, socially, or in terms of employability. It is in these circumstances that choices often need to be made, and depending on those choices different outcomes, some good and some bad, will result. It is then that patients may become more conscious of the dominance of the voice of restitution in the illness narratives told by health care providers, and how difficult it can be to get their own questing voice heard and their chaotic voice acknowledged.

I am not referring simply to the possibility that when patients make their wishes clear and unequivocal that they may be ignored or persuaded to subsume them to the will of the doctor. Although such paternalism undoubtedly exists, I am here more interested in the potential for a failure of communication to occur when health care providers speak with the voice of the restitution narrative and patients with the voice(s) of the quest and / or chaos narrative(s).

13. The Constructed Nature of Ethical Discourse

Applying Frank's analysis to the nature of the different voices present in the narratives medical ethicists tell, the following claims can be made about the nature of the voices in these narratives.

The voices are culturally constructed such that those wishing to tell or to enact stories have available to them a variety of ways of telling them, or voices to tell them through, depending on their cultural background.

These off-the-peg voices are different in different cultures. They are specific to but not exclusive to different cultures at different times.

The narrative voices in this case are specific to contemporary medical ethicists.

There are structural differences between the voices of the different narratives.

14. What Does this Mean in Practice?

To explain what this might mean in practice let us consider what might happen under ideal circumstances when the voice of restitution is dominant in the clinical encounter. Ideally, the values of the patient will be highly influential in the way in which the health care provider chooses to frame that narrative of restitution, and this framing will then lead to the development and delivery of a system of health care that recognises and acknowledges these values. It may be that the system pays inadequate attention to some of the things that the patient values, such as how to live with the chronic consequences of illness, but at least the system will address those aspects of the patient's condition that are both amenable to cure and that the patient cares about.

Now let us consider a real situation in which despite all attempts to achieve this ideal something far from ideal resulted. The situation involves the delivery of prenatal counselling to British Muslim women at risk of giving birth to babies with the severe genetic condition thalassaemia. As a result of a misunderstanding by health care professionals about the choices that this group of women would or would not make when faced with the results of screening, a considerable number of women were simply not offered screening, either in time for it to be feasible for them to request a termination of pregnancy or at all. It provides a powerful example of what can happen when the dominant narrative of restitution fails to reflect the values of the patient, and when the relative subordination of the patient's quest narrative makes it difficult to materially alter the nature of the dominant narrative.[10]

Another example of this is available through the personal account of a woman with sickle cell disease.[3] Sickle cell disease is an inherited condition that, amongst other things, makes pregnancy very hazardous for those affected. Since pregnancy entails great danger to women with sickle cell disease, the voice of the restitution narrative might well counsel against becoming pregnant. For this particular woman, however, having a child is an important life goal and one for which she is willing to countenance the risk of ill health and even death. The woman describes her frustration at the health care system's apparent inability to appreciate that a woman with sickle cell disease might wish to actively contemplate pregnancy. She is counselled about contraception and she is told about the risks of pregnancy, but no one discusses the real if slim possibility of a successful pregnancy. Despite the fact that a successful pregnancy, with both mother and child well, is less likely for a women with sickle cell disease, for this woman at least, the chance to explore the possibilities of pursuing this part of her life journey is an important one.

I would argue that getting your voice heard as a patient is made more difficult by the relative weakness of the voice of the quest narrative in the health care encounter. As Foucault argued so cogently[1] when reading a text it is incumbent on the reader to try and understand what is not said as well as what is said, and to try and understand who is empowered to speak and who is not. I would argue that the dominance of the voice of the restitution narrative in encounters between patients and health care professionals reflects the power relationship between these two parties. Health care professionals are in a powerful position in these encounters: the voice of the restitution narrative that they favour is dominant and it is easier for professionals than for patients to speak and to be heard.

15. Why Any of this Matters

One explanation of the dominance of the voice of restitution in the illness narrative told by doctors is the problem solving focus of medical education and training. Medical students are taught, from an early age, to identify problems (diagnose) and find solutions (prescribe treatments). Order is actively sought, chaos is equated with failure, and patients learn to live with their illness, with little or no acknowledgement by the medical system that the illness experience has any meaning beyond the (hopefully) temporary deviations in normal function it imposes. For example, when a woman's breast cancer is fully excised, and she remains disease free for five years, she is considered cured: the problem has been solved, and according to the medical narrative she has been restored to health. The patient's narrative is not so straightforward and linear. It involves chaos as she is faced by her fears, and the fears of her family and friends. The extent to which she experiences this chaos is dependant on many factors, including her own experience of breast cancer, the existence of other serious illnesses amongst her family and friends, the way in which her own sense of identity is dependent on her bodily integrity, and the way in which, culturally, the story of those with breast cancer is constructed.

Ethical discourse, like clinical practice, involves the application of problem solving skills, in this case reasoning, to the ethical dilemmas faced by patients, families, doctors, and society. This is not a method that welcomes chaos but rather, like the medical approach, seeks to create order and objectivity: a problem is identified, a solution is found, the problem is solved. Patients however do not experience ethical dilemmas in their lives as linear problems that cease to concern them once they've independently, or with help, submitted the identified area of concern to methodical moral reasoning: for example, parents still agonise years afterwards about the decision to terminate pregnancies incompatible with life outside the womb,[26] or to opt for pregnancies considered by doctors, statistically, too risky to pursue.

16. Conclusion

An enhanced appreciation of the context within which illness is experienced and of the highly constructed and inter-subjective nature of moral reasoning offers a practical and challenging way to think about pressing contemporary ethical issues in medicine. If moral imperatives are to have meaning for those they affect then the rich complexities of the language through which ethical debates are conducted, the conceptual realities of patients, families, professional carers and society, and the context within which we all make decisions, will need to be acknowledged by ethicists and incorporated into the stories they tell. Much of the philosophical reasoning about the ethical issues raised by the practice of modern medicine is of course a solitary pursuit, undertaken by individual patients, by family members, by professional carers, or by philosophers far removed from the practical task of clinical care. Nevertheless, whether ethical examination takes place in a public arena or in private contemplation, the search for meaning is an underlying objective and is conducted by all of the players in this ethical debate.

Notes

[1] M Foucault, *The history of sexuality: volume 1, an introduction*, Penguin, London, 1990, p. 27.

[2] D Kirklin, 'The role of the humanities in the education and support of physicians delivering palliative care', in D Doyle, G Hanks, N Cherny and K Calman (eds), *The Oxford Textbook of Palliative Medicine*, 3rd edition, Oxford University Press, Oxford, 2003, pp.1182-1189.

[3] D Kirklin, 'The New Genetics: retelling and reinterpreting an old story', in M Evans and I Finlay (eds), *Medical Humanities*, BMJ Books, London, 2001, pp. 101-118.

[4] D Kirklin, 'The Altruistic Act of Asking', in *J Medical Ethics* 2003, 29, pp. 193-195.

[5] M Foucault, *Birth of the clinic: an archaeology of the human sciences*. Trans. A M S Smith, Routledge, London, 1976, p. 8.

[6] D Kirklin, 'Diabetes and stem cells: a guide to the ethical debate', *Br J Diabetes Vasc Dis*, 2, 2002, pp. 198-201.

[7] A McIntyre, *After virtue: a study in moral theory*, 2nd Edition, Duckworth, London, 1981.

[8] B Williams, 'Persons, character, morality', in B Williams, *Moral luck*, Cambridge University Press, New York, 1981, pp. 1-19.

[9] RS Downie, 'Supererogation and altruism: a comment', in *J Med Ethics*, 28, 2002, pp. 75-76. Robin Downie has suggested that an alternative to using moral reasoning to persuade doctors to behave in certain ways might be to enshrine what were formerly seen as the moral duties of doctors in their formal terms of employment. To paraphrase Williams, by doing so we would be in danger of leaving little opportunity for those generous and genuine acts of kindness, giving, and sharing of humanity that give meaning to medicine, including anything that could inspire doctors to take any moral goal seriously. Will the result be doctors following the letter of their contract but, ultimately, less committed to the spirit of the moral goals written so carefully into it? Current developments in relation to the employment contracts for general practitioners and hospital consultants in the UK suggest that this may indeed be an unwelcome consequence of such an approach.

[10] D Kirklin, *Poetry, pictures, and the sexual demographics of health.* In M Worton and N Tagoe-Wilson (eds), *Our national healths*, Cavendish Press, London, 2004, pp. 211-219.

[11] Aristotle examined the aspects of a man's character that made him good. What exactly would feature on such a list of virtues is debateable but might for instance include courage, compassion, self-control and patience. This ancient idea, that there are certain qualities or virtues that are morally praiseworthy, was re-visited by Elizabeth Anscombe in GEM Anscombe, 'Modern moral philosophy', *Philosophy*, 33, 1958, pp. 1-19. Anscombe argued that the historical notions of morality made no sense in the modern world and that without a lawgiver it makes no sense to live by laws. She argued that the dissociation between the origin of the prevailing moral laws and their role in everyday life resulted in virtue becoming an end in itself, unrelated to human needs or desires. She called for a return to an examination of the qualities, both virtues and vices, which describe the types of character we might admire. Alasdair MacIntyre (see reference 12) took Anscombe's analysis further, arguing that modern societies had

inherited a hodgepodge of ethical traditions and that this inevitably led to moral confusion. He called for a revival of an Aristotelian account of human good which would ground a modern set of virtues and provide a meaningful context for the lives people lead.

[12] D Kahneman and A Tversky, 'Choices, Values, and Frames', *American Psychologist*, 39, 1984, pp. 341-50.

[13] A Tversky, D Kahneman, 'Rational choice and the framing of decisions'. J of Business; 59, S251-S278, 1986, p. 209.

[14] D Kreps, *Notes on theory of choice*. Westview Press, London, 1988, pp. 196-7.

[15] J Nash, 'The bargaining problem', *Econometrica,* 18: 2, 1950, pp. 155-162.

[16] M Osborne and A Rubinstein, *A course in game theory,* MIT Press, London, 1994, pp. 209-219.

[17] The prisoner's dilemma was designed by Merrill Flood and Melvin Dresher in 1950, as part of the Rand Corporation's investigations into game theory. The dilemma involves two accomplices in a crime who are each offered the opportuntiy to confess their crime. They cannot consult with each other and indeed do not even know if they are both being offered the same deal. The conundrum for each of the prisoners is this: each is better off confessing than remaining silent, but if both confess then each of them is worse off than if they had both remained silent. The prisoner's dilemma has spawned many research papers and fired the imagination of scholars from a variety of disciplines including mathematics, economics and philosophy. For a detailed history of the prisoner's dilemma see S Kuhn, 'Prisoner's Dilemma', in *The Stanford Encyclopedia of Philosophy (Fall 2003 Edition)*, Edward N. Zalta (ed.), http://plato.stanford.edu/archives/fall2003/entries/prisoner-dilemma Accessed 4th August 2004.

[18] K M Hunter, *Doctors' stories: the narrative structure of medical knowledge*, Princeton University Press, Princeton, NJ, 1991, pp. 3-26.

[19] H Brody, 'My story is broken: can you help me fix it?', in *Literature and Medicine* 13, 1, 1994, pp. 79-82.

[20] D Kirklin, 'Metaphors for medicine: revealing reflections or just popular parodies?', in *J Medical Ethics: Medical Humanities* 27, 2001, p. 89.

[21] D Kirklin, 'Foreword', in *The Oncologist*, 7, Supplement 2, 2002, pp.1-2.

[22]. Narratologists working within literary theory have a range of differing views on what narrative is. It is beyond the scope of this chapter to review these different views in any detail.

[23] A Frank, 'Reclaiming an orphan genre: the first-person narrative of illness', in *Literature and medicine*, 13, 1,1994, pp. 1-21.

[24] Despite important cultural differences between North America and the UK, the narrative voices described by Frank are clearly discernible both in UK clinical practice and in UK patient narratives.

[25] C Saunders, 'Foreword', in D Doyle, G Hanks, N Cherny and K Calman (eds), *The Oxford Textbook of Palliative Medicine,* 3rd edition, Oxford University Press, Oxford, 2003, pp. 1182-1189.

[26] Making difficult decisions: 'A child of mine', a video made by the Child Bereavement Trust 2000, provides a powerful first-hand account of the ethical crisis faced by parents offered a termination of pregnancy for fetal abnormality incompatible with life.

Bibliography

Anscombe, E., 'Modern moral philosophy'. *Philosophy*, 33, 1958.

Brody, H., 'My story is broken: can you help me fix it?'. *Literature and Medicine* 13, 1, 1994.

Downie, R.S., 'Supererogation and altruism: a comment'. *J Med Ethics*, 28, 2002'

Foucault, M., *The history of sexuality: volume 1, an introduction*. Penguin, London, 1990.

Foucault, M., *Birth of the clinic: an archaeology of the human sciences*. Translated by A M S Smith, Routledge, London, 1976.

Frank, A., 'Reclaiming an orphan genre: the first-person narrative of illness'. *Literature and medicine*, 13, 1, 1994.

Kahneman, D. and Tversky, A., 'Rational choice and the framing of decisions'. *J of Business*; 59, 1986.

Kahneman, D. and Tversky, A., 'Choices, Values, and Frames'. *American Psychologist*, 39, 1984.

Kirklin, D., 'Poetry, pictures, and the sexual demographics of health'. M Worton and N Tagoe-Wilson (eds), *Our national healths*, Cavendish Press, London, 2004.

Kirklin, D., 'The role of the humanities in the education and support of physicians delivering palliative care'. D Doyle, G Hanks, N Cherny and K Calman (eds), *The Oxford Textbook of Palliative Medicine*, 3rd edition, Oxford University Press, Oxford, 2003.

Kirklin, D., 'The Altruistic Act of Asking'. *J Medical Ethics*, 29, 2003.

Kirklin, D., 'Diabetes and stem cells: a guide to the ethical debate'. *Br J Diabetes Vasc Dis*, 2, 2002.

Kirklin, D., 'Foreword'. *The Oncologist* 7, Supplement 2, 2002.

Kirklin, D., 'The New Genetics: retelling and reinterpreting an old story'. M Evans and I Finlay (eds), *Medical Humanities*, BMJ Books, London, 2001.

Kirklin, D., 'Metaphors for medicine: revealing reflections or just popular parodies?'. *J Medical Ethics: Medical Humanities* 27, 2001.

Kreps, D., *Notes on theory of choice*. Westview Press, London, 1988.

McIntyre A., *After virtue: a study in moral theory*. 2nd Edition, Duckworth, London, 1981.

Making difficult decisions: 'A child of mine'. Video made by the Child Bereavement Trust 2000.

Nash, J., 'The bargaining problem'. *Econometrica*, 18: 2, 1950.

Osborne M. and Rubinstein A., *A course in game theory*. MIT Press, London, 1994.

Hunter, K. M., *Doctors' stories: the narrative structure of medical knowledge*. Princeton University Press, Princeton, NJ, 1991.

Saunders C., 'Foreword'. D Doyle, G Hanks, N Cherny, and K Calman (eds), *The Oxford Textbook of Palliative Medicine*, 3rd edition, Oxford University Press, Oxford, 2003.

Williams, B., 'Persons, character, morality'. *Moral luck*, Cambridge University Press, New York, 1981.

Dialogue and Creativity – Narrative in the Clinical Encounter

Jan C. Frich

Abstract

This chapter discusses recent developments within the field of 'narrative-based medicine'. The main argument is that the concept of 'healing dramas' captures essential aspects in the clinical encounter, and supplements the approach in which the patient is conceptualized as 'text'. The healing drama offers conceptual tool that helps us to understand processes in which narratives are performed in clinical settings. This approach reveals the active role physicians also have as producers and co-authors of 'text' in clinical encounters. The chapter is centred on a narrative that has been constructed on the basis of the author's own clinical experience as physician at a department of neurosurgery. The narrative is analysed and discussed by using a multi level approach to narrative put forward by the physician and philosopher Howard Brody in his book *Stories of sickness*. The chapter will highlight the hermeneutic character of diagnostic reasoning in clinical medicine, and particularly discusses the tension between 'cases' and 'dramas'. The chapter discusses how insights Mikhail Bakhtin's theory of the polyphonic novel can help us to conceptualise the clinical encounter as a genuine dialogue in which 'healing dramas' emerge.

Key Words: doctor-patient-relationship; narrative; patient; text

*****

> '[W]e were far too concerned with 'defectology', and far too little concerned with 'narratology', the neglected and needed science of the concrete'. Oliver Sacks (1985)

Patients repeatedly construct and tell stories about their experiences with illness. These stories are embedded in broader life-stories that again influence how each individual understands and copes with illness. These stories do not emerge in a vacuum, rather illness narratives are informed by scripts and plot structures that make sense within a particular culture. As suggested by the vast literature on narrative and illness, the meaning of illness must be understood as both a personal and social phenomenon.[1] Narrative plays a key role in how medical knowledge is constructed and applied in health care settings.[2] Medical journals have published articles that address the importance of narrative in relation to health and illness.[3] Theories of 'narrative medicine' and 'narrative-based medicine' have been put forward and discussed in several recent books.[4] One might propose that 'a narrative turn' has emerged within medicine.

1. 'The Patient as Text'

A central assertion within narrative-based medicine is that human action can be analysed as text.[5] Stephen L. Daniel was probably the first who suggested conceptualising the patient as a 'text'.[6] The 'text' in question is, however, a very complex phenomenon that can be 'read' on many different levels: as the human body, the patient's story, the physician's construction of diagnostic meaning, the management of treatment, and as related to the patients' sense of being healed.[7]

One may argue that there is a fundamental difference between interpreting a more or less stable text compared with studying the patient's story or the dialogue of a clinical encounter.[8] Furthermore, a patient's story rarely constitutes a coherent narrative that the physicians can easily interpret or read. Illness narratives are more likely to appear as 'fragmentary', 'fragile', and to be characterized by their unstable and changing meanings.[9] There is also a danger in focusing too much on the *patient* as textual entity, and consequently overlooking the active role physicians also have as producers of texts about the patient. The implication of this critique is that the text in clinical medicine should not be considered as a stable object, but as a dynamic process shaped by those who take part in the clinical encounter.

2. Plot

A narrative plot configures one story out of multiple events: it organises events in time, and it organises different components, such as unintended circumstances, discoveries, chance, and unintended results.[10] Paul Ricoeur claims that human experience is characterized by a 'pre-narrative' quality, and that narrative plays a central role in the processes which negotiate personal identity.[11] Ricoeur proposes three frameworks for understanding the relation between life and narrative. First, the logic of human action and narrative is similar. Human beings act intentionally, and in this sense, we understand ourselves and our actions in ways which are similar to how we interpret agents in a literary universe. Humans think in terms of projects, aims, means, and circumstances, and this 'conceptual network of human action' is structured in ways that echoes the order of the literary plot. Second, human actions are 'readable'; they can be interpreted and retold by means of signs and rules, similar to those of literary narratives. Finally, Ricoeur claims, life involves a 'search,' 'a 'quest,' or a 'demand' for narrative. Throughout the life of a human being, various processes will necessarily bring about series of events such as illness and suffering that require a search or a quest for narrative.

3. 'Healing Dramas'

Time occupies a central role in narrative. Literary critic, Frank Kermode, uses the distinction between *chronos* and *kairos* to help explain how time is managed and represented in literary plots. While *chronos* refers to 'waiting time' or 'passing time', *kairos* signify moments of crisis between a beginning and an end which represent 'a point in time filled with significance, charged with a meaning derived from its relation to the end'.[12] A characteristic of literary plots is that they often focus on crisis and endings; their organization of events therefore often transgresses and escapes *chronos* and instead reflects primarily the logic of *kairos*.

Cheryl Mattingly makes use of the distinction between *chronos* and *kairos* when arguing that not all moments in clinical practice are equally filled with 'narrative significance'. In certain situations very much may be at stake for the ones involved, and these moments can turn out to be 'more narrative,' and hence more kairos, than others.[13] Mattingly claims that at such moments in the clinical encounter narratives can be *acted* or *performed* in what she refers to as 'healing dramas' or 'performance narratives'.[14] Healing dramas 'involve the active shaping of present moments' and thus play a powerful role in the clinical encounter.[15] The concept of the healing drama captures essential aspects in the clinical encounter that are easily overlooked. The healing drama helps conceptualising the process in which narratives are performed and the active role physicians may have as producers of 'text'.

I will first present Mohammad's story, which I have constructed based on my own clinical experience. Based on this story, I will highlight the hermeneutic character of diagnostic reasoning in clinical medicine, and then point to the tension between 'cases' and 'dramas'. I will then analyse Mohammad's story by using a multilevel approach to narrative proposed by Howard Brody. Finally, I suggest that Mikhail Bakhtin's theory of the polyphonic novel and dialogic model might provide important insights for understanding the central role of the physician's creativity in a clinical encounter

4. Mohammad

Mohammad, a thirty-five year old man, is admitted to hospital with an acute, severe headache, vomiting and neck stiffness. The CT-scan gives us the diagnosis 'subarachnoid hemorrhage' (a live-threatening bleeding from an artery on the surface of the brain). He is feeling sick and has thrown up

twice. He looks anxious, and it is difficult for me to make him cooperate. He does not speak Norwegian, but I get the impression that he understands that he has a bleeding inside his head and that it is a serious condition. We decide not to perform any operative procedures. We observe him over night at the intensive care unit and start medical treatment.

'Mohammad wants you to turn his bed around so that it points towards Mecca'. His cousin serves as interpreter.

'He would like pray'. This is not an easy operation in an intensive care unit (the place is crowded with severely ill patients and there is technological equipment everywhere; he has a urine catheter, infusion kits, the monitors).

'You have a serious condition and you should be resting in your bed', I say to him and think to myself: 'His blood pressure is far too high, if he goes on like this we may need to give him sedatives to calm him down'. But he insists on praying. He accepts lying in bed if we help him turn the bed towards Mecca. Finally, we agree do the best we can. After a while Mohammad talks with his cousin who turns to me asking: 'Mohammad wonders if this bleeding can be caused by thinking very much?'

'Thinking ... thinking very much?' What a strange question, I think to myself. Is this some kind of cultural phrase for something I do not know about? I ask: 'What does he actually mean by that?'

'Doctor, he has been very concerned with the situation in our home country lately. I know he is awake at night sometimes. He is anxious about our family, and he worries about our future', his cousin explains.

How should I respond to this? I say: 'Well, to the extent that thoughts and worries raise the blood pressure, there may be an association. If his concerns have caused stress which again raises the blood pressure, this may have caused the wall of his artery in his head to rupture'.

I watch him carefully as his cousin translates what I have said. As his cousin talks he appears to be calmer, and then ... then he looks at me with a thankful expression of his face.

5. The 'Case' in Medical Hermeneutics

The first task of clinical medicine is to listen to the patient, to assess symptoms and findings, and to make an interpretation. Oliver Sacks has put it this way:

> The patient presents his 'story' with a naive immediacy and force – this is what he has been experiencing, been feeling; the physician (it is hoped!) listens not just sympathetically but *knowledgeably*, with a knowledge of other 'cases', and of the physiological and pathological processes of the

> organism, which he is able to correlate, creatively, with what the patient is telling him.[16]

In order to make a diagnosis, to recognize the patient as a 'case', the physician must have general knowledge about diseases. The physician must also have acquired skills in clinical reasoning, which involves practical knowledge about the associations between clinical signs and diseases. This knowledge constitutes the basis from which a physician can make a decision about which interpretation, out of all possible interpretations, that is most likely true in a particular case.

The story about Mohammad illustrates how the physician's interpretive skills are used in a diagnostic process in which a 'case' is inferred from a clinical reality. Mohammad's complaints, symptoms and bodily dysfunction (headache, nausea, and neck stiffness) and pathological findings (CT-scan) – *signs* – are indications (symptoms) of an abnormal bodily process (intracranial bleeding) – *object* – which the physician associate with a specific disease which enables him to make a diagnostic inference (subarachnoid hemorrhage) – *interpretation.* This triadic relation between signs, objects, and interpretations represents the core in clinical, diagnostic reasoning.[17] The example illustrates how clinical medicine involves hermeneutic or semiotic processes. One point needs to be underlined; interpretations are made when all three components are being dealt with. What a physician sees as a sign in a given clinical context is a product of interpretations which are informed by theories about symptoms. Likewise, an inference between a set of signs and an abnormal bodily process is informed by theories about how certain signs are indicators of such processes. A diagnosis represents the final product of this interpretive process. In a seminal article, Roland Barthes has described this hermeneutical character of clinical medicine:

> … disease is in fact made intelligible as a person who is first of all in the body's secret, under the skin, if I may say so, and who emits signs, messages, which the physician must receive and interpret rather like a deciphering soothsayer: this is, in reality, a divination, a mantic art.[18]

In Mohammad's case the diagnosis was established through a rather straightforward interpretive process. In other cases the physician may have problems with concluding diagnostically about the patients' symptoms and bodily dysfunction. In some cases there may be a high degree of uncertainty and disagreement about the interpretation of signs.

6. Cases and Dramas

While the diagnostic act recognizes the patient as a 'case,' the clinical case has a purely medical focus which excludes the personal experience of illness.[19] According to Oliver Sacks, we must deepen the case history to a narrative or a tale in order to get an understanding of the patient as subject. We must learn about 'the experience of the person, as he faces, and struggles to survive, his disease'.[20] In serious neurological disease, Sacks argues, a personal drama will unfold: 'A *world* is lost or broken or unmade, reduced to bits and pieces, to chaos – and it is a *world*, no less, that must be remade'.[21] In order to help the patient, the physician would often need access to the patient's lifeworld.

In Mohammad's case, the diagnosis 'subarachnoid hemorrhage' represents a medical interpretation of a set of clinical signs, but this interpretation also turns into a new sign for the patient. The patient now asks himself what this sign, the diagnosis, means in terms of *cause* ('why me, why now?'), *prognosis* ('am I likely to survive this?'), *personal meaning* ('what does this mean to me and how does it influence my life?'), and *management* ('what can be done about it?'). Owing to these unanswered questions, Mohammad's story illustrates a moment filled with narrative significance

Illness often involves some form of 'biographic disruption'.[22] Arthur W. Frank has observed that illness narratives often convey some sense of 'being shipwrecked by the storm of disease' and at a moment in the narrative the patient can best be described as a 'narrative wreck'.[23] Mohammad probably feels that his world has been reduced to 'bits and pieces': he has been thrown into a 'narrative wreck'. This is the state from which he invites the physicians to help him in his struggle to construct a meaningful illness-narrative. To use Frank's metaphor, the construction of narrative becomes a way of doing repair work on the 'narrative wreck'.[24] This is the situation in which a healing drama emerges.

7. Multilevel Narrative Analysis

Howard Brody claims that physicians encounter narratives at four levels: the first, level is constituted by patients' stories of their episodes of illness, the second, by patients' life stories from which they seek to make sense of their illness episodes, the third,involves the cultural prototypes for stories that makes sense within a society, and finally, the last level includes the overarching narratives or 'sacred stories' designed to situate adherents of a belief system within human history and the larger cosmos.[25] In examining the healing drama that emerges in the encounter between Mohammad and his physician, we will rely on Brody's typology.

His illness episode probably provides Mohammad with 'a sense of an ending'[26], in which a moment of narrative significance, a sense of *kairos,* emerges as he tries to make sense of the chaotic situation he finds himself in. In so doing, he tries to construct a meaningful illness narrative, and the implicit and explicit negotiation of emplotment, or the *causal* ordering of events, and *personal meaning ascribed to them, becomes significant.,*

Let us suppose that Mohammad felt his illness was a result of some sort of divine punishment. Had he failed in his belief? Had he sinned? When being faced with a potentially deadly condition, one must assume that questions such as these became of crucial importance to him. In order to find answers, Mohammad turns to his God to consult the divine narrative voice, an act that illustrates Brody's 'sacred' level. But perhaps Mohammad was certain that the episode did not represent a punishment for violating sacred rules, and that he instead examines his life in order to find alternative explanations as to what might have caused the episode? Viewed from such a 'life story' level, Mohammad hypothesizes that his thoughts and worries may have played a role. Has his bleeding been caused by too much thinking? He also invites the physician to comment on this alternative plot. At first, in accordance with the 'cultural prototype' level, the physician had interpreted Mohammad's question as rather unusual. By asking him to explain what he meant, the physician realizes that the patient literally is talking about 'stress'. Had the mental pain caused damage in his brain? The physician's reply provides Mohammad with the necessary bits of information and authority that makes t possible for him to construct an alternative, meaningful explanation of his illness episode. This final interaction illustrates Brody's 'illness narrative' level.

The outcome of this healing drama constitutes a coherent illness narrative which makes sense within Mohammad's life story, and which maintains, or perhaps strengthens, his personal identity. The narrative allows Mohammad to link his personal suffering with the grand narrative about the situation of his family and his home country. He is now able to see himself as a *victim*, but at the same time as a *hero*: as someone who had been wounded in a mental struggle for his family, his home country, his values and beliefs.

The application of Brody's levels to Mohammad's story, points to the importance of personal, social and cultural contexts in understanding an illness narrative. In such analysis, it is often necessary to reflect on what constraints a narrator may face or what motives he or she may have when constructing a specific narrative.[27] The limitation of this approach is that what is said is often a result of what *can* be said in a specific context. Sometimes it can be more important to reflect on what is *not* said, given a certain context, than what is explicitly articulated.

8. Dialogue and Polyphony

Paul Ricoeur claims that an important difference between life and fictional narratives relates to the question of authorship:

> [W]e learn to become the *narrator* and the *hero of our own story*, without actually becoming the *author of our own life*. We can apply to ourselves the concept of *narrative voices* .... We can become our own narrator, in imitation of these narrative voices, without being able to become the author.[28]

Ricoeur's perspective reminds us of the limited agency of the individual patient in 'the patient as text.' The events that cause the illness have often been brought about by forces outside the individual's own control, and in a sense one can say that the true 'author' of the text is represented by the disease or life itself. This 'author', however, is resisted and contested by the therapeutic actions of the patient and his or her social environment (which also involves the physician). What a patient or a physician can do to help the patient gain agency is to provide a 'narrative voice' to the processes that take place in the patient's body. In this limited sense one may apply the concept of authorship, or perhaps co-authorship, to both the patient and the physician.

If we see the clinical encounter as a drama between at least three different actors, as exemplified by the patient, the disease, and the physician, it becomes clear that the encounter will be characterized by more than one voice. Elliot G. Mishler draws attention to this by speaking about 'the voice of medicine' and 'the voice of the lifeworld'.[29] If we think of communication as a transmission of signs that give meaning within a particular system of signification, we can also speak about the 'voice of the disease'. This voice manifests itself through the patient's symptoms. Schematically, we can say that while the voice of medicine is centered on diagnosis and medical treatment, that the voice of the lifeworld represents the patient's interpretation of the disease, or his or her values, which help form the quest for a meaningful illness narrative. The complexity of the encounter and the number of voices increase if we include the patient's family members, other health professionals, etc. Each speaks from different positions and perspectives.

Mikhail Bakhtin's concept of 'polyphony' might provide a significant perspective for understanding the complexity of a clinical encounter. In *Problems of Dostoevsky's poetics* Bakhtin claims that literary critics have characterized Dostoevsky's novels as 'chaotic' and as 'a conglomerate of alien materials and incompatible principles of design'.[30] The reason for this, he argues, is that critics read Dostoevsky's novels as if they were written as 'monologic' novels. They expect to find *one* authoritative voice that reflects the unified consciousness, the 'Weltanschauung', of a single author. Instead Bakhtin claims that Dostoevsky's novels are *dialogic* and thus break with the narrative organization and implicit world view of the monologic novel. According to Bakhtin, Dostoevsky lets his characters speak for themselves, and as a result his novels are characterized by a variety of equal narrative voices:

> The plurality of independent and unmerged voices and consciousnesses and the genuine polyphony of full-valued voices are in fact characteristics of Dostoevsky's novels. It is not a multitude of characters and fates within a unified objective world, illuminated by the authors unified consciousness that unfold his work, but precisely the plurality of equal consciousnesses and their worlds, which are combined here into the unity of a given event, while at the same time retaining their unmergedness.[31]

If we apply Bakhtin's theory of the 'polyphonic novel' to the clinical encounter, dialogue, perspective and polyphony emerge as central concepts. In a clinical encounter the patient and the physician probably view certain things in a similar mode the unique place each of them occupies in the situation, there will always be aspects of the situation that the two of them view differently. The ideal clinical encounter should not always be based on the merging of different voices. What Bakhtin's concept of 'polyphony' can help us acknowledge, is that the clinical encounter will always involve *different* voices, and perspectives, as well highlight that there are different things at stake for the different participants. If one expects to find a monologic order, the clinical encounter may appear what Bakhtin refers to as 'a conglomerate of alien materials and incompatible principles of design'[32]. An alternative model for understanding the clinical encounter is therefore the polyphonic dialogue, in which different voices can be articulated and different perspectives recognized. In contrast, however, to Dostoevsky's polyphonic novels, the clinical encounter has a pragmatic aim: while Dostoevsky's literary characters can refrain from merging their voices or seeking agreement, the patient and the physicians need to establish some kind of shared understanding that can form the basis for therapeutic action.

Rather than consisting of a free flux of polyphonic perspectives, a clinical encounter requires some degree of negotiation between different voices and different stories. From the physician's point of view not all plots are feasible, not all stories are possible. Some stories are, medically speaking, better than others. These narrative 'constraints' may be based on medical knowledge, professional experience, professional ethics, and the organizational, political, financial and juridical context. Similarly, the patient will also perceive some stories as better than others. Polyphonic encounters are precisely characterized by allowing such diverging opinions and narratives. From a polyphonic perspective, disagreements between patients and physicians can be understood as conflicts about narrative authority, and the physician has a particular obligation to acknowledge that there are many ways to tell a story.

9. Conclusion

The narrative metaphors involved in the healing drama captures essential aspects in the clinical encounter are difficult to identify when operating with the objectifying notion of the 'patient as text'. In contrast, a dialogic approach to the healing drama helps us acknowledge the significance of performativity to the narrative processes of the clinical encounter, and therefore also the active role physicians play in these processes as producers of 'text'. I have tried to demonstrate that there is an inherent tension between 'cases' and 'dramas' in clinical medicine. Physicians may be able to pay more attention to the literary and narrative aspects of the clinical medicine if they adopt a dialogic model for the clinical encounter.

Notes

1 A Kleinman, *The illness narratives: suffering, healing and the human condition*, Basic Books, New York, 1988. A W Frank, *The wounded storyteller: body, illness, and ethics*, University of Chicago Press, Chicago, 1995. C Mattingly, 'Emergent narratives', in C Mattingly and L C Garro (eds), *Narrative and the cultural construction of illness and healing*, University of California Press, Berkeley, 2000, pp. 181-211. B Hurwitz, T Greenhalgh, V Skultans (eds), *Narrative research in health and illness*, Blackwell, Oxford, 2004.

2 K M Hunter, *Doctor's stories: the narrative structure of medical knowledge*, Princeton University Press, Princeton, NJ, 1991.

3 R Charon, 'Narrative medicine: form, function, and ethics', in *Annals of Internal Medicine*, 134, 2001, pp. 83-87. M F McLellan and A H Jones, 'Why literature and medicine?', in *Lancet*, 348, 1996, pp. 109-111. T Greenhalgh and B Hurwitz B, 'Why study narrative?', in *British Medical Journal*, 318, 1999, pp. 48-50.

[4] R Charon, *Narrative medicine: honoring the stories of illness*, Oxford University Press, Oxford, 2006. T Greenhalgh and B Hurwitz (eds), *Narrative-based medicine: dialogue and discourse in clinical practice*,.BMJ Books, London, 1998. T Greenhalgh, *What seems to be the trouble? Stories in illness and healthcare*, Radcliffe Publishing, Oxon, 2006. K Montgomery, *How doctors think: clinical judgement and the practice of medicine*, Oxford University Press, Oxford, 2006. J Launer, *Narrative-based primary care: a practical guide*, Radcliffe Medical Press, Oxon, 2002. F Rapport and P Wainwright (eds), *The self in health and illness: patients, professionals and narrative identity*, Radcliffe Publishing, Oxon, 2006.

[5] P Ricoeur, 'The model of the text: meaningful action considered as text', in *Hermeneutics and the human sciences*, Cambridge University Press, Cambridge, 1981, pp. 197-221.

[6] S L Daniel, 'The patient as text: a model of clinical hermeneutics', in *Theoretical Medicine*, 7, 1986, pp. 195-201.

[7] ibid.

[8] R Ahlzén, 'The doctor and the literary text – potentials and pitfalls', in *Medicine, Health Care and Philosophy*, 5, 2002, pp. 147-155.

[9] L J Kirmayer, 'Broken narratives: clinical encounters and the poetics of illness experience', in C Mattingly and L C Garro (eds), *Narrative and the cultural construction of illness and healing*, University of California Press, Berkeley, 2000, pp. 153-180.

[10] P Ricoeur, 'Life in quest of narrative', in D Wood (ed), *On Paul Ricoeur: narrative and interpretation*, Routledge, London, 1991, pp. 20-33.

[11] Ricoeur, 'The model of the text: meaningful action considered as text', Ricoeur, 'Life in quest of narrative'.

[12] F Kermode, *The sense of an ending: studies in the theory of fiction*, Oxford University Press, Oxford, 1967, p. 47.

[13] C Mattingly, 'Performance narratives in the clinical world', in B Hurwitz, T Greenhalgh, and V Skultans (eds), *Narrative research in health and illness*, Blackwell, Oxford, 2004, pp. 73-94.

[14] ibid., and C Mattingly, *Healing dramas and clinical plots: the narrative structure of experience*, Cambridge University Press, Cambridge, 1998.

[15] Mattingly, 'Performance narratives in the clinical world', p. 74.

[16] O Sacks, 'Clinical tales', in *Literature and Medicine*, 5, 1986, p. 16.

[17] J Nessa, 'About signs and symptoms: can semiotics expand the view of clinical medicine', in *Theoretical Medicine*, 17, 1996, pp. 363-377. J D Johansen and S E Larsen, *Signs in use: an introduction to semiotics*, Routledge, London, 2002.

[18] R Barthes, 'Semiology and medicine', in *The semiotic challenge*, Basil Blackwell, Oxford, 1988, pp. 202-213.

[19] W F Monroe, W L Holleman, M C Holleman, 'Is there a person in this case?', in *Literature and Medicine*, 11, 1992, pp. 45-63.

[20] O Sacks, *The man who mistook his wife for a hat*, Picador, London, 1985, p. x.

[21] Sacks, 'Clinical tales', p. 18.

[22] M Bury, 'Chronic illness as biographical disruption', in *Sociology of Health and Illness*, 4, 1982, pp. 167-82.

[23] Frank, *The wounded storyteller: body, illness, and ethics*, p. 54

[24] ibid.

[25] H Brody, *Stories of sickness*, Oxford University Press, Oxford, 2003.

[26] Kermode.

[27] M Bury, 'Illness narratives: fact or fiction?', in *Sociology of Health & Illness*, 23, 2001, pp. 263-285.

[28] Ricoeur, 'Life in quest of narrative', p. 32.

[29] E G Mishler, *Research interviewing: context and narrative*, Harvard University Press, Cambridge Mass., 1986, 142-143.

[30] M Bakhtin, *Problems of Dostoevsky's poetics*, Ardis, Ann Arbor, 1973, p. 5.

[31] ibid., p. 4.

[32] ibid., p. 5.

Bibliography

Ahlzén, R., 'The doctor and the literary text – potentials and pitfalls'. *Medicine, Health Care and Philosophy*, 5, 2002, pp. 147-155.

Bakhtin, M., *Problems of Dostoevsky's poetics*, Ardis, Ann Arbor, 1973.

Barthes, R., 'Semiology and medicine'. *The semiotic challenge*, Basil Blackwell, Oxford, 1988, pp. 202-213.

Brody, H., *Stories of sickness*. Oxford University Press, Oxford, 2003.

Bury, M., 'Chronic illness as biographical disruption'. *Sociology of Health and Illness*, 4, 1982, pp. 167-82.

Bury, M., 'Illness narratives: fact or fiction?'. *Sociology of Health & Illness*, 23, 2001, pp. 263-285.

Charon, R., 'Narrative medicine: form, function, and ethics'. *Annals of Internal Medicine*, 134, 2001, pp. 83-87.

Charon, R., *Narrative medicine: honoring the stories of illness*. Oxford University Press, Oxford, 2006.

Daniel, S.L., 'The patient as text: a model of clinical hermeneutics'. *Theoretical Medicine*, 7, 1986, pp. 195-201.

Frank, A.W., *The wounded storyteller: body, illness, and ethics*. University of Chicago Press, Chicago, 1995.

Greenhalgh, T. and Hurwitz, B. (eds), *Narrative-based medicine: dialogue and discourse in clinical practice*. BMJ Books, London, 1998.

Greenhalgh, T. and Hurwitz, B., 'Why study narrative?'. *British Medical Journal*, 318, 1999, pp. 48-50.

Greenhalgh, T., *What seems to be the trouble? Stories in illness and healthcare*. Radcliffe Publishing, Oxon, 2006.

Holquist, M., *Dialogism: Bakhktin and his world*. 2. ed. Routledge, London, 2002.

Hunter, K.M., *Doctor's stories: the narrative structure of medical knowledge*. Princeton University Press, Princeton, NJ, 1991.

Johansen, J.D. and Larsen S.E., *Signs in use: an introduction to semiotics*. Routledge, London, 2002.

Kermode, F., *The sense of an ending: studies in the theory of fiction*. Oxford University Press, Oxford, 1967.

Kirmayer, L.J., 'Broken narratives: clinical encounters and the poetics of illness experience'. Mattingly, C. and Garro, L.C. (eds), *Narrative and the cultural construction of illness and healing*, University of California Press, Berkeley, 2000, pp. 153-180.

Kleinman, A., *The illness narratives: suffering, healing and the human condition*. Basic Books, New York, 1988.

Launer, J., *Narrative-based primary care: a practical guide*. Radcliffe Medical Press, Oxon, 2002.

Mattingly, C., *Healing dramas and clinical plots: the narrative structure of experience*. Cambridge University Press, Cambridge, 1998.

Mattingly, C., 'Emergent narratives'. Mattingly, C. and Garro, L.C. (eds), *Narrative and the cultural construction of illness and healing*, University of California Press, Berkeley, 2000, pp. 181-211.

Mattingly, C., 'Performance narratives in the clinical world'. Hurwitz, B., Greenhalgh, T., and Skultans, V. (eds), *Narrative research in health and illness*, Blackwell, Oxford, 2004, pp. 73-94.

McLellan, M.F. and Jones, A.H., 'Why literature and medicine?'. *Lancet*, 348, 1996, pp. 109-111.

McLellan, M.F., 'Literature and medicine: narratives of physical illness'. *Lancet*, 349, 1997, pp. 1618-1620.

Mishler, E.G., *Research interviewing: context and narrative*, Harvard University Press, Cambridge, Mass., 1986.

Monroe, W.F., Holleman, W.L., and Holleman, M.C., ''Is there a person in this case?''. *Literature and Medicine*, 11, 1992, pp. 45-63.

Montgomery, K., *How doctors think: clinical judgement and the practice of medicine*. Oxford University Press, Oxford, 2006.

Nessa, J, 'About signs and symptoms: can semiotics expand the view of clinical medicine'. *Theoretical Medicine*, 17, 1996, pp. 363-377.

Rapport, F. and Wainwright, P. (eds), *The self in health and illness: patients, professionals and narrative identity*. Radcliffe Publishing, Oxon, 2006.

Ricoeur, P., 'The model of the text: meaningful action considered as text'. *Hermeneutics and the human sciences*, Cambridge University Press, Cambridge, 1981, pp. 197-221.

Ricoeur, P., 'Life in quest of narrative'. Wood, D. (ed), *On Paul Ricoeur: narrative and interpretation*, Routledge, London, 1991, pp. 20-33.

Sacks, O., *The man who mistook his wife for a hat*. Picador, London, 1985.

Sacks, O., 'Clinical tales', In *Literature and Medicine*. 5, 1986, pp. 16-23.

Clinical Tales and the Artlike Creativity of the Body

Drude von der Fehr

Abstract
'Is any fusion of the biological and historical possible?' The British neurologist Oliver Sacks asks in his article 'Clinical Tales', and this is one question which lies at the heart of any study of literature and medicine. I maintain in this chapter that aesthetic theories often rely on implicit biological, or more precisely, psychological paradigms. The question of whether there is an artlike lifeworld, therefore similarly invokes questions of the possible relations between a notion of aesthetic immediacy and theories of brain development. With these questions in mind, I explore how it is to live in a world that we can call aesthetic. I argue that to live a 'style,' or to live in the world of art, however, might induce pain in that it involves a potential loss of biological capacity. I also want to suggest that an examination of the aesthetic lifeworld in the framework of biological or psychological theories, might propose new hypothesises in medical theory. In my exploration, I take as my starting point, two clinical tales by the Russian neuropsychologist Aleksandr Romanovich Luria (1902-1977).

Key Words: Neuropsychology; to live a style

*****

The question of the possibility of a fusion between the biological and the historical, interested A. R. Luria throughout a lifetime. Oliver Sacks, a most ardent follower of doctor Luria, states in his forword to the 1987 edition of Luria´s *The Man with a Shattered World* that he 'was the most significant and fertile neuropsychologist of his time and raised neuropsychology to a subtlety and simplicity which could not have been imagined fifty years ago'. (Luria's studies are based on the presumption that the functions of the brain are only partly biological and that we must understand any patient, be it a stroke victim or an amputee, as a human being trying to cope with the human condition in an existential sense, rather as someone suffering merely from 'a medical condition' Illness therefore constitutes part of a phenomenological, or aesthetic lifeworld, which conventional medicine has erased by reducing the experiences of the suffering person to a medical diagnosis. The psychologist Jerom S. Bruner understands Luria as arguing that 'the explanation of any human condition is so bound to context, so complexly interpretive at so many levels, that it cannot be achieved by considering isolated segments of life...'.[1] A phenomenological approach to illness is important, also in the cases in which medical science has been the most insistent on its biological paradigm, such as in the medicical approaches to illnesses that relate to our cognitive functions. The thought that our brain functions were not wholly biological and that any brain damage must be studied contextually, is central to the understanding of Luria's concept of 'romantic science.' Luria's insistence on the necessity of studying illness contextually, will therefore constitute a significant focus in my exploration of his two clinical tales.

1. What is 'Romantic Science'?

'Romantic science' is a central concept to Luria's invention of what we can call a new genre of medical writing.. Instead of ordinary case-stories with their focus on anatomical and phsysiological facts, Luria wrote biographical narratives. Sacks calls these clinical tales. According to Ann Hunsaker Hawkins, Luria's clinical tales constitute narratives that 'would give expression to scientific reality by resorting to devices of literary form'.[2] Hawkins here alludes to the biographical, life-story form of the clinical tale. A clinical tale treats an illness in relation to treatment, but since an illness does not exist apart from an ill person, a clinical tale must involve a 'retrospective consideration of a life [3].'[4] Oliver Sacks, for instance, defines clinical tales as:

> 'clinical' insofar as they have a factual, clinical basis, and lend themselves to a clinical or medical analysis. And they are 'tales' insofar as they have a subject – and a theme – neither of which is possessed by a description or case history.[5]

Clinical tales introduce or re-introduce the subject at a deeper and existential level[6] and delineates how worlds may be broken, or buffeted by disease, and how these worlds may be organized anew and transformed by deeply alien experiences.[7] The introduction of the themes of identity and world-experiences, is to doctor Sacks 'indispensable for medical understanding, practice, and communication.'[8] In commenting on A. R. Luria's and Oliver Sacks' notion of clinical tales, Kathryn Montgomery Hunter suggests in *Doctor's Stories* that:

> Medical as they are literary, these cases set the standard for physicians' full empathic and analythical narratives of illness and treatment. They were conceived as antidotes and

> supplements to the standard case history so as to embody their authors' enrichment and extension of their medical fields.[9]

Clinical tales involve the doctors as much as the patients. In this sense they constitute a double perspective: the clinical tale includes both the story of the doctors' changing understanding and their empathic engagement with the patients' experience, and the suffering patients' struggle to maintain a self and to re-organize his or her life-world. Thus clinical tales focus on the particularity of each patient as well as of the particular dialogic process between the doctor and the patient which takes place in their co-operative interpretation of the disease and in the therapeutic strategy that is being worked out.

2. The Mind of a Mnemonist

One of Lurias'clinical tales tells the story of a man with an exeptional memory, the mnemonist, S., whose mind had been structured to accommodate his superior mnemic ability.[10] His exceptional capacity was virtually without limit, and his memory 'functioned in such a way that any verbal cue would immediately evoke a rich and complex set of eidethic and syneasthetic imagery. For example, a given word (or sound) would not only be instantly converted into a visual image, but would also evoke other senses, such as taste or smell.'[11] We can easily imagine what an effort it was for S. to read, when each word evoked powerful synaesthetic imagery. His memory functioned in a literal, metaphorical mode: S. walked in the colors, shades and sounds of his memory, where all of his experiences were kept intact.

Even in his childhood, this synaesthetic mode had made S. into a dreamer. As a result, S. became passive. The overwhelming sense impressions paralyzed him. Instead of being able to act, S. was acted upon. The lively impressions of his memory make him into a man who was always waiting for something great to happen to him. In addition to his lively, synaesthetic memory, S. developed an ability to 'see' himself as an image of another person who carried out his instructions. This was an enormous help to S. in regulating his behavior. For example, Luria describes how 'he could control his vegetative processes and eleminate pain by transferring it to another person.'[12] In time, however, when his mnemic capacities had been even more sharpened, S. experienced a tendency to digress, which made it hard for him to keep track of a topic in conversation. About S.'experience of reality and family life, Luria concludes:

> He had a family – a fine wife and son who was a success – but this, too, he perceived as though through a haze.

> Indeed, one would be hard put to say which was more real for him: the world of imagination in which he lived, or the world of reality in which he was a temporary guest.[13]

The inner life of S. must have seemed more real to him, than any external reality.

3. Qualitative Immediacy

Owing to S.' synaesthetic memory, he lived in a world without the secure structures of epistemology. Instead, he was doomed to exist in a world characterized by 'qualitative immediacy.' The philosophy of the American pragmatist John Dewey might help illuminate this concept. Dewey's concept of aesthetic experience, as he outlines it in *Art as Experience*, is preceisely characterized by qualitative immediacy. According to Dewey, art is not located in the object itself. Instead, art is constituted in the body of the maker and/or in the body of the perceiver. But qualitative immediacy does not mean that we can experience art directly and unmodified through sense-impressions only.[14] Instead Richard J. Bernstein insists that the 'struggle to give proper due to immediacy is the backbone of Dewey's theory of experience and nature':

> Dewey attempted to disentangle the important recognition of the pervasiveness of immediacy from the mistaken claim that there is immediate *knowledge*. A good slogan for Dewey's view would be: Qualitative immediacy – Yes! Immediate knowledge – No![15]

Immediate qualities are had or felt, but not known. They are the consequences of intelligent, that is inferential, perceptual action on all levels of interaction between human organism and its environment. As such, immediate qualities are had or felt by the mind/body.

S. was a dreamer who was lured by the intensity of his own images to believe them true. The mnemonist therefore actually lived in a world of aesthetic immediacy. This is a biological fact. In the actual world, S. always appeared to be waiting for something particular to happen. While waiting, however, the only action that would take place would primarily be located in his synesthetic imagination. In this sense S. lives in an artlike world. The implications for literary studies are intriguing. Does the example of S. suggest that it is possible to live the world of art? If so, in which ways could this influence medical thinking? In the following section I argue that the particularity of an artlike world and the connection between language, metaphorical experience and the brain challenges conventional medical thinking.

4. On the Track of the 'Essence of the Unique in Romantic Science'

The Man with a Shattered World, the other clinical tale of Luria, was based on 25 years of observation and on 3000 pages of autobiographical notes made by a brain damaged patient, Zazetsky. Zazetsky was shot in the head during World War II. *The Man with a Shattered World* is a result of the doctor's editing of Zazetsky's autobiographical notes. Together, *The Mind of a Mnemonist,* based on 30 years of observation and experiments, and *The Man with a Shattered World,* constitute classics in the clinical literature on pathologies of memory. However, the cases which are described differs, widely. While the memory of the mnemonist retains everything and he as a consequence is forced to live in a world of estehtic immediacy, Zazetsky's dysfunctional memory functions in the opposite manner.

Before I examine the case of Zazetsky, I will, however, explain the concept of 'romantic science.' According to Bruner, it is in the final chapter of Luira's autobiography that he provides a clearer definition of this concept. In his definition, Luria poses 'romantic science' against what he calls 'classical science.' While classical science formulates general laws, romantic science seeks, 'neither to split living reality into its elementary components nor to represent the wealth of life's concrete events in abstract models that loose the properties of the phenomena themselves.'[16] In constrast to the classical method, romantic science points to the importance of context and of 'the essens of the unique' in neurological studies. According to Luria, the writing of neurological case-studies as biography differs qualitiatively from classical science's study of general laws in that such (auto)biographical case-studies include the individual context of each disease or brain injury. Luria emphasizes these individual contexts in relation to the study of neurological disorders because they help retain 'the properties of the phenomena themselves.'[17] The significance Luria ascribes to a phenomenologiocal approach is illustrated by how he introduces the last chapter of his autobiography by quoting Goethe: 'Gray is all theory; green grows the golden tree of life.' (Jerome S. Bruner, Forword to the 1987 edition of *The Mind of the Mnemonist*) Neurologists must, according to Luria, supplement their classical scientific approach by attempts to identify the inner laws of each event, which reflect the uniqueness of each event in its setting.[18] '

5. The Importance of the Particular

What, more precisely, does searching for the 'essence of the unique' involve? First, one must identify, as far as I can see, the essential problem of each case. Instead of focusing on the essence of the damage, one must look for the essentials in the patient's identity-formation and lifeworld. One significant question in identifying the implications for the patient's lifeworld involves posing questions, such as: what is the essence of the trouble that the damage causes for the patient? When this is answered, one will have gained significant knowledge about the probable function of each particular damage or disease. This process also involves making inductive inferences which might help us form new and fruitful hypothesises. While nomothetic reasoning (seeing each case as an example of a general law)[19] is most common in medicine, the discourse of 'romantic science' aims at establishing new hypothesises. This endavour can be likened to the function of poetic language and its ability to fight the doxa or automaticity in language. In this sense, there exists a close kinship between the medical discourse of romantic science and poetic language or art. Therefore, I propose that there is indeed a connection between biology and humanistic diciplines.

In the case of the mnemonist, is not his world of immediate qualities both a poetic world and a world of the essences of each particular phenomenon? Each particular thing has its taste, sound and image. However, existing in a qualitative world like this, involves difficulties, not only with teleological action, but also with representative thinking.

6. The Man with a Shattered World as Autobiography

In reading *The Man with a Shattered World* as an autobiography, one must aknowledge that autobiography in itself does not unproblematically provide an unmediated represention of the somatic body in literary discourse. As a genre, autobiography does not provide a self-evident link between biology and history, but is rather, according to James Olney, characterized by its claim to a specific ontology. This special order of reality, or ontology, is closely associated with the timespan of the *bios* (the life) of auto-bio-graphy. An autobiography will also always contain the following question: How is that which is no longer living going to be restored to life?[20] An autobiography will therefore somehow have to address the question of memory, and in so doing it will have to question the role of consciousness in the actualization of lost facts. Implied in the ontology of autobiography is that the 'bios' is joined by a dual I: the present narrator and the past, narrated self. Consciousness' role is to hold together in memory the I who remembers and the I who lived the life remembered. Olney proposes 'that the term *bios* simultaneously ... is both the course of a life seen as a process rather than a stable identity and the unique psychic configuration that is this life and no other.'[21] Autobiography is close to life in the sense that it thematizes the process of time and the actual consciousness involved in the writing of this memory, but on the other hand it might be highly fictitious because factual memory might be weak and forgetfulness might indeed be very creative.[22]

Autobiography does, however, always combine the question of identity and world-experience.

7. Zazetsky's Struggle

The writing of autobiography always involves a construction of identity, and identity is again always in a certain sense a fiction. Zazetsky, the man with the severe brain damage caused by the bullet wound, experiences, however extraordinary difficulties in constructing his identity. Owing to his condition, he lacks a permanent self from which to write his identity, and therefore his attempted discursive transactions with former and younger selves becomes fundamentally destabilized. Zazetsky's world is in a constant state of flux and he constantly perceives the world as one constituted by a shifting, visual chaos. His memory, language and thought becomes dysfunctional. He cannot even remember his own bodily functions: When he wants to defecate, he cannot remember his anus.[23] Zazetsky cannot remember his former life, nor can he conceive of a psychic configuration that is unique to him, and this is precisely Zazetsky's main problem: he struggles with his lifeworld, which appears shadowy, dreamy and without any appearance of reality.

Thanks to his writing, however, Zazetsky in time experiences that his condition changes. The aim of his struggle is, according to himself, to find a way to live, not merely to exist.[24] It is difficult, if not impossible, to have the feelings of living being, without having some concept of oneself. The strive for an identity is thus a strive for a feeling of existence and a liveable lifeworld. But in order to live or to make a lifeworld, one also needs the fiction of a self or at least the process that leads towards such a configuration.

8. The Curative Side of The Man with a Shattered World

As an autobiography *The Man with a Shattered World* is outstanding. In it a narrator, a doctor, has taken the place of the self constructing itself. The historical A. R. Luria is of course not identical with the doctor in the text, but it is nevertheless this doctor-narrator, and not Zazetsky himself, who narrates Zazetsky's identity. To himself, Zazetsky remains only a name. He never successfully manages to construct an identity, though the writing functions as a way to *try* to hold together a world which has fallen into fragments. In spite of suffering from severe brain damage, Zazetsky he retains the capacity for self-evaluation (since this specific function of the brain was not damaged). Luria, the narrator, says that Zazetsky's immediate grasp of the world was spared, as well as his will, desire and sensitivity to experience, thus allowing him to evaluate each failure.[25] This explains how it was possible for him to restore a more coherent memory and how he could engage in a process of figuring a self through autobiographical writing.

In the text the doctor-narrator acts as a guarantor, or a permanent perspective, in the process of identity formation. Identity is always dialogical, normally we both see ourself from the outside, and from the inside, that is, as memories of former selves. In this case Zazetsky needs the gaze of the doctor in order to work on stiching together his memory-fragments. Zazetsky improves gradually: verbally he can stich together more and more memories, but when he dies, his experiences of himself is still fragmented. It is only after Zazetsky's death that Luria's narrative provides him with a life as a coherent, individual person Thus, the narrator's account gives Zazetsky an identity which is authorized by the historical Luria when he published the book in 1968..

One does not need a literary approach to acknowledge the curative side of the clinical tale. *A literary interpretation, however, underlines this aspect of the text.* If every engagement with a patient is therapeutical, as well as diagnostical, clinical tales describe not only othe facts of the actual damage, but help the patient to a useful, however fictitious, identity. Luria thought that inventions of language and culture led to an unfolding of unsuspected potentialities in man and that mind grows by the incorporation of cultural and historical innovation (Bruner 1987). The therapeutical side of autobiographical writing lies in the fact that it helps the mind evolve and in that autobiography has a restorative biological as well as an existential effect. By enlarging the mind and understanding of both the patient and the doctor, an autobiographical, literary approach can have the potential to heal. Thus, literary interpretation can help the body act creatively.

9. A Postmodern Self in Biological Life

The story of Zazetsky is more than an an autobiography. The self-evaluation and fragmentation characteristic of Zazetsky's verbal effort to construct a self, is also typical of the postmodern novel. Zazetsky works on forming an identity, but there is no stable phenomenological framework towards which he can turn his mind. There is only flux and fragmentation. As a result, there is no way that Zazetsky can know himself. Thus, he appear as scepticism biologically embodied. The gaze from the outer world is the only guarantee he has of existing as a coherent being.

According to Brian MacHale, modern fictions are preoccupied with epistemology, while postmodernistic fiction focuses on ontology.[26] This is also the case in autobiographical novels. In the case of Zazetsky's autobiography, it refuses the possibility of any foundation of knowledge. It does not address epistemological questions. There is no possible foundation for establishing a coherent self in Zazetsky's notes. The self in these notes lacks any epistemological foundation, just as the postmodern fictional selves. The story of Zazetsky represents a postmodern groundless prosess of self, in pathological reality. The quest for identity is wholly an ontological matter. Even though Zazetsky does not inhabit what we normally conceive of as an identity, he has retained the urge and the self-reflection necessary *to want to become one*. But how can the process towards identity start when there is no ground to start from? Is it possible to have a self, or a process towards a self, without any memory of a former self that serves as the foundation of consciousness?

10. Being Expresses Itself

Umberto Eco discusses 'primary indexicallity' in the chapter 'On Being' in his book *Kant and the Platypus* (1997). He states that first we have a reaching out towards something (which one also can call a desire). This 'something' has the status of a possibility. But in order for it to come into being, this reaching out towards a possibility, must be articulated.[27] Luria, the narrator, suggested that Zazetsky had an immediate grasp of reality, but in order to make himself real, also for himself in his ability to self-evaluation, Zazetsky must verbalize something which he can call himself. Thus, it looks, as if we can only have a process towards establishing a self with the help of language. About the relationship between language and self, the American philosopher Vincent Colapietro says in his article, 'Striving to Speak in a Human Voice: A Peircean Contribution to Metaphysical Discourse':

> Think here of the later Martin Heidegger's claim regarding our relationship to language: while it is correct to say that humans speak, it is so superficial as to be misleading. For a language speaks and humans only speak in response to having been addressed by language. Whatever sort of instrument language might be, it is not the sort of instrument we can pick up and put down. It is so intimately a part of our selves that Charles S. Peirce's assertion is, when properly qualified, more plausible than not: 'my language is the sum total of myself'. My language, however, is never simply mine; it overwhelmingly belongs to us, that is, some historically evolved and evolving community. My language is, at once, 'there,' existing apart from me in the habits and artifacts of others, and 'mine,' something existing as part of me.[28]

Language takes hold of me. And this 'something' that holds me together, is me.

At first there was for Zazetsky a frantic struggle for words.[29] This frantic struggle stops when the doctor suggests a method of automathical writing. It turns out that spontaneously Zazetsky can write whole words and sentences. He does not *remember* how to write. His ability to write has the appearance of spontaneously being there, of ontology. By approaching Zazetskys' efforts we are approaching questions of being or ontology. The ability to write is central to Zazetsky's quest, it comes to him spontaneously as a sort of ontological ground. Zazetsky is this ontological ground, and his self is also a struggle to become a self in time and space. This, striving to become a 'bios,' is a fictional discourse. As Nietzche holds in *Ecce Homo,* the creation of a self is always a fictional phenomenon. But it starts from Being struggling to express itself.

Postmodern *style* is perhaps also preoccupied with ontology? In reading Zazetsky's story with an emphasis on style, the similarities with postmodernist fictions emerge. The novels and drama of the Norwegian writer, Jon Fosse, exemplifies a similar preoccupation with 'being' without the security of any epistemology.

As suggested previously, through poetic language, history can have a direct effect on biology. The creative, innovative language of poetry might perhaps have a special influence on the 'growth of the mind'? The French Professor in Literary Studies, Gérard Danou, quotes, in a paper on the surrealist author, Henri Michaux, J-M Rey who states that the language of the poet emerges from a body that does not want to yield to the every-day nature of knowledge that is supposed to be contemporary with him.[30] Language emerges from the body, but it creates a fictional self which both represent a wish to accomodate itself to doxa, and the self fights against 'the most ordinary and most aberrant effects of some of our knowledge.'[31] In striving to piece together a language which could express his being, Zazetsky's quest is similar to the poet's. He is struggling to become an epistemologically based self, while at the same time language itself takes ove and makes Zazetzky a poetic, postmodern self, a being in becoming. To live such a style – the becoming of a self – is indeed painful, just as living in a universe without representation or epistemology can be associated with existential, or even, physical pain.

11. Pathologies of Style?

As exemplified by Luria's *The Man with a Shattered World*, there seems to exist certain pathologies of style. Because such styles express the existential circumstances of human life, the effects caused by such styles might therefore often be experienced as painful. While these pathologies of style reflect external conditions, such as existential, epistemological or ontological ones, they are also found in verbal fictions. Literary, pathological styles, however, must not be understood as direct effects of an author's disease. The relation between discursive style and the patient's pathology is not a matter of a simple, mechanistic model of cause and effect.. Instead, literary styles express creative actions, and function therefore as configuations of a theme.[32] Although these styles might have a therapeutical function, the case of Zazetsky also clearly illustrates that the healing of Zazetksy's cognitive functions as well as the discourse of of his autobiography were orchestrated by his doctor Styles are in this sense verbal creations which have external effects on both readers and writers. Thus both Zazetsky and Luria were affected by the writing *The Man with a Shattered World.*

12. The Embodiment of Language

> Luria was convinced that the aim of mental functioning was to construct two complementary versions of the same world. Indeed, he urged that the human nervous system is structured in a manner to help us achieve this dual representation and to help us put the two representations together.' One version was a simultaneous world, the other a temporally organized world, structured around plans and intentions. Importantly he thought that language plays a crucial role as mediator between the two worlds and the two functions of the brain.[33]

Luria approach implies that language has a biological function. In *The Man With a Shattered World* Luria states: '[a]part from being a means of communication, language is fundamental to perception and memory, thinking and behavior. It organizes our inner life'.[34] Luria therefore suggests that language has to do with the ontological 'something' which we call 'us'.

In his latest book on autobiography *How Our Lives Become Stories* (1999), Paul John Eakin introduces cognitive science in the study of autobiography. He refers to the neurobiologist and Nobel-laureate, Gerald M. Edelman, who with his 'neural Darwinism' articulates a theory of the way in which the brain's neural organization is constantly modified to adapt to changing demands of experience'.[35] Brain events are active and represent constructions made by the individual organism.[36] According this view, the brain is authentically one's own and indeed unique. Thus, Luria's romantic science seems to have been a precursor of the cognitive science of today.

Modern cognitive science[37] sees language as part of the body, and as a consequence, everyday communication is understood as constituted by processes taking place in the mind/body. Language is a result of the embodiment of the organism, as well as of unconscious and metaphorical thought. Reason and our sense of what is real depends crucially upon our bodies, 'especially our sensorimotor apparatus, which enables us to perceive, move, and manipulate, and the detailed structures of our brains, which have been shaped by both evolution and experience'.[38] Human beings think in categories, and categories are made unconsciously and metaphorically in experience.

Zazetsky struggled to find a language and to organize himself into a person. After the accident, language in this sense was no longer available to Zazetsky, and he was forced to recover it. Because of this loss, Zazetsky's experiences of himself and the world changed greatly. With the loss of his language, and he had also 'lost' part of his body. Zazetsky could, for example, not remember his left side, and constantly struggled to stich together a memory of something he could no longer experience. Zazetsky tried to recall something which no longer had any experimental validity to him. Even if he remembered a word, the fact that he had 'lost' his left side, made it difficult for him to experience the basic metaphorical structure of language, and thus made the word, 'left,' incomprehensible. Even more significant, the damage seems to have caused a loss of Zazetsky's mental body-schemata. Though the acquisition of language had a therapeutical effect in the way that his mind and cognitive functions gradually were restored, the world could not become real to Zazetsky unless he made for himself a language which was based on his new experiences. In order to make himself a new language, Zazetsky needed a new mental picture of his body.

The essence of the unique case of Zazetsky, is partly explained by his aphasia. Zazetsky could only make the therapeutical effort of categorizing for himself a liveable life through remaking an embodied form of thinking and language, but he never got that far. His brain never healed enough to make it possible for him to form the hypothesises necessary to recreate such a new world for himself. His struggle to form a new language made his cognitive functions develop, but not enough for Zazetsky to ever leave the painful state of postmodernity.

13. Conclusion

The reading of Luira's two neurological tales suggests that 'romantic science' implies a somatic aesthetics in that they illustrate that the physical body, both artistically and medically, can function as a site for creativity. The partial healing of Zazetsky shows how a somatic reality can function in ways that are analogous to art. Both Zazetsky and S. exist in an artlike world. While Zazetsky, inhabit a postmodern world, S. lives in a world of immediate aesthetic experience. Both these worlds, despite their eventual beauty, are fundamentally 'unreal,' and therefore experienced as painful and confusing.

Luira's clinical tales also clarifies the importance of hypothesis-making in medical discourse. The quest for the ability to reason in these tales, also suggests that a world without epistemology hurts. Postmodernism's emphasis on the ontological and lack of concern for the epistemological (Brian McHale 1989, Pöstmödernist Fiction: 10), seems to be deeply pessimistic in the sense that it represents a loss of human capacity, also in the sense of biological capacity. However, postmodernism also represents a hope of growth, both in terms of bodily capacity and of cognitive reasoning. Thus, both postmodernism and art as a whole are deeply ambivalent. While they both might be associated with pain, they also represent the potential of growth, both of the somatic body and of medical scientific discourse.

Notes

[1] Jerome Bruner 2002, 'Forword' to the 1987 edition of *The Mind of a Mnemonist* by A.R.Luria.)

[2] A H Hawkins, 'A.R. Luria and the Art of Clinical Biography', in *Literature and Medicine* 5, 1986, p. 2.

[3] ibid., p. 2.

[4] ibid., p. 3.

[5] O Sacks, 'Clinical Tales', in *Literature and Medicine,* 5, 1986, p. 16.

[6] ibid., p. 17.

[7] ibid., p. 18.

[8] ibid., p. 16.

[9] K M Hunter, *Doctor's Stories*, 1991, p. 164.

[10] A H Hawkins, 'A.R. Luria and the Art of Clinical Biography', p. 6.

[11] ibid., p. 7.

[12] A R Luria, *The Mind of a Mnemonist.* Harvard University Press, Cambridge, Massachusetts and London, 2002, p. 154.

[13] ibid., p. 159.

[14] I allude here to an article I have written, Fehr, D.v.d., 'Art et Instinct' in *Questions de sémiotique,* A. Hénault, D. Savan, D.v.d. Fehr and J.-C. Pariente (eds). Presses Universitaires de France, Paris, 2002.

[15] R J Bernstein, *John Dewey*, Washington Square Press, Inc., New York, 1967, p. 92.

[16] Jerome S. Bruner 2002, 'Forword' to the 1987edition of *The Mind of a Mnemonist*

[17] Jerome S. Bruner 2002, 'Forword' to the 1987edition of *The Mind of a Mnemonist*

[18] Jerome S. Bruner 2002, 'Forword' to the 1987edition of *The Mind of a Mnemonist*

[19] A H Hawkins, 'A.R. Luria and the Art of Clinical Biography', p. 6.

[20] J Olney, 'Some Versions of Memory/Some Versions of Bios: The Ontology of Autobiography' in *Autobiography. Essays Theoretical and Critical*, Princeton University Press, Princeton, New Jersey, 1980, p. 237.

[21] ibid., p. 241.

[22] ibid., p. 262.

[23] O Sacks, 'Clinical Tales', in *Literature and Medicine,* 5, 1987.

[24] ibid., p. 17.

[25] A R Luria, *The Man with a Shattered World.* Harvard University Press, Cambridge, Massachusetts, 1997, p. 33.

[26] B McHale, *Postmodernist Fiction*, Routledge, London and New York, 1987, p. 9.

[27] U Eco, *Kant and the Platypus*, A Harvest Book, San Diego, New York, London, 1997, p. 22.

[28] V Colapietro, 'Striving to Speak in a Human Voice: A Peircean Contribution to Metaphysical Discourse', *The Review of Metaphysics*, 58, December 2004, p. 372.

[29] Jerome S. Bruner 2002, 'Forword' to the 1987edition of *The Mind of a Mnemonist*

[30] G Danou, 'Henri Michaux in Search for his *Tempo* or Great Health'. Paper held at the conference, 'Illness in Context', Oslo 27.-29 October 2004, p. 11.

[31] ibid., p. 11.

[32] See the Norwegian Professor in Comparative Literature, Kjersti Bale, in her book of 2003, *Tekstens Tempering*, where she argues for a special style in Montaignes essay.

[33] Jerome S. Bruner 2002, 'Forword' to the 1987 edition of *The Mind of a Mnemonist*

[34] A R Luria, *The Man with a Shattered World*. Harvard University Press, Cambridge, Massachusetts, 1997, p. 33.

[35] P J Eakin, *How Our Lives Become Stories*, Cornell University Press, Ithaca and London, 1999, p. 13.

[36] ibid., p. 17.

[37] G Lakoff and M Johnson, *Philosophy in the Flesh*, Basic Books, New York, 1999.

[38] ibid., p. 17.

Bibliography

Bernstein, R. J., *John Dewey*. Washington Square Press, Inc., New York, 1967.

Colapietro, V., 'Striving to Speak in a Human Voice: A Peircean Contribution to Metaphysical Discourse'. *The Review of Metaphysics*, 58, December 2004, p. 367-398.

Danou, G., 'Henri Michaux in Search for his *Tempo* or Great Health'. Paper held at the conference, 'Illness in Context', Oslo, 27.-29 October 2004.

Dewey, J., *Art as Experience*. The Berkley Publishing Group, New York, 1980.

Eakin, P.J., *How Our Lives Become Stories*. Cornell University Press, Ithaca and London, 1999.

Eco, U., *Kant and the Platypus*. A Harvest Book, San Diego, New York, London, 1997.

Fehr, D.v.d., 'Art et Instinct'. *Questions de sémiotique,* A. Hénault, D. Savan, D.v.d. Fehr and J.-C. Pariente (eds), Presses Universitaires de France, Paris, 2002.

Hawkins, A.H., 'A.R. Luria and the Art of Clinical Biography'. *Literature and Medicine* 5, 1986.

Hunter, K.M., *Doctor's Stories*. Princeton University Press, Princeton, New Jersey, 1991.

Jakobson, R. and Halle, M., *Fundamentals of Language*. Mouton Publihers, The Hague, Paris, New York, 1980.

Lakoff, G. and Johnson, M., *Philosophy in the Flesh*. Basic Books, New York, 1999.

Luria, A.R., *The Man with a Shattered World*. Harvard University Press, Cambridge, Massachusetts, 1997.

Luria, A.R., *The Mind of a Mnemonist*. Harvard University Press, Cambridge, Massachusetts and London, 2002.

McHale, B., *Postmodernist Fiction*. Routledge, London and New York, 1987.

Olney, J., 'Some Versions of Memory/Some Versions of Bios: The Ontology of Autobiography'. *Autobiography. Essays Theoretical and Critical*, Princeton University Press, Princeton, New Jersey, 1980.

Sacks, O., 'Clinical Tales'. *Literature and Medicine,* 5, 1986, pp. 16-23.

Signs of Illness

Vincent Colapietro

Abstract
There is, at the center of the various contexts in which illness must be situated in order to be understood (above all, the archeological, the phenomenological, and clinical contexts) a reflexive task. That is, there is the task of interpreting our practices of interpreting the signs of illness (at least, that of assembling the materials for such an interpretation). In my own investigation of this task, I am oriented by the conception of illness as an alteration in *our comportment toward the world.* Hence, illness is, first and foremost, a modification of our orientation toward the everyday. The relevant phenomena – the most salient ways in which illness *shows* (or announces) itself – are in effect somatic signs, *broadly conceived:* the manifest intimates the latent, the perceptible insinuates the hidden, but this occurs in reference to what Maxine Sheets-Johnstone calls intercorporeality, not only (not even primarily) in reference to the body either in isolation from others or in abstraction from its engagements with the world. The investigation of illness in this and indeed any other legitimate sense depends, above all else, on the complex interplay between two dynamic factors – the free play of the theoretical imagination and a fidelity to the disclosures of experience. The discourses of medicine as well as those of literature can contribute to both of these factors. Both do so not least of all by exposing the unsuspected limitations and distortions inherent in our habitual or customary frames of meaning. They expose these limitations and distortions by suggesting alternative frames, rival schemes, of intelligibility. The movement back and forth from wider to narrower spheres of significance is a mark of intellectual vitality and health, whereas the inability to move from more restricted to more encompassing contexts – and back again – is a symptom of intellectual illness. Even more radically, illness and literature can expose the dulling or deadening of sensibility that results from a tyrannical preoccupation with significance, a stultifying fixation on intelligibility.The final conclusion to which we are led in this provisional investigation (hence, only a provisionally final conclusion) is this. The most pathological frameworks of interpretation are precisely those that occlude the *fateful paradoxes of illness* in their irreducibly paradoxical and uniquely fateful character. Literature is especially effective in making visible these occlusions, in exposing this pathology of interpretation.

Key Words: Philosophy and pragmatism; semiotics and medicine.

> Considering how common illness is, how tremendous the spiritual change that it brings, how astonishing, when the lights of health go down, the undiscovered countries that are then disclosed, what wastes and deserts of the soul a slight attack of influenza brings to view, what precipices and lawns sprinkled with bright flowers a little rise of temperature reveals, what ancient and obdurate oaks are uprooted in us by the act of sickness, how we go down into the pit of death and feel the waters of annihilation close above our heads and wake thinking to find ourselves in the presence of the angels and the harpers when we have a tooth out and come to the surface in the dentist's armchair and confuse his 'Rinse the mouth – rinse the mouth' with the greeting of the Deity stooping from the floor of Heaven to welcome us – when we think of this, as we are so frequently forced to think of it, it becomes strange indeed that illness has not taken its place with love and battle and jealousy among the prime themes of literature. – Virginia Woolf, 'On Being Ill'

1. Introduction

Paradoxically, contextualizing illness entails wresting it from the abstract discourse in which it has been traditionally situated (i.e., from the discursive 'context' in which thick descriptions of the variable sites of human illness are mostly absent). Archeology, phenomenology, and the clinic identify three concrete contexts especially worthy of exploration, not least of all because each one has the power to expose just how thin and abstract have been so many traditional conceptualizations of human illness. Moreover, there is, at the center of each of these contexts, a reflexive task: that of interpreting our practices of interpreting the signs of illness (at least, that of assembling the materials for such an interpretation). But this reveals the relevance of both semiotics and hermeneutics to the task of adequately contextualizing illness. An understanding of these practices relies, however implicitly and unsystematically, on an understanding of the functioning of signs and the work of interpretation. In light of this, the immensity and complexity of the task of understanding *illness in context* would be hard to exaggerate.

Let me begin, nonetheless, with an *archeological* point, one concerning the origin (or *arché*) of the practice of interpreting the signs of illness. The history of medicine and that of semiotics are intertwined, so intimately and early that the art of healing was to a significant degree defined in terms of the art of interpreting somatic signs as indications of health, disease, and recovery.[1] Clearly, diagnosis and prognosis are most effectively made by those possessing the art (or *techné*) of discerning the significance of perceptible bodily changes (the art of taking this cluster of alterations to mean the likelihood of this disease).

But this brings us immediately to a *phenomenological* point: illness *manifests itself* somatically. Diagnoses, treatments, and prognoses are authorized and assessed in reference to these manifestations. More generally, part of the meaning of illness is to be disclosed by painstaking descriptions of the lived experience of embodied agents. (There is nothing inherently or invincibly subjective about this experience: phenomenology does not attend to subjective experience but rather strives to be faithful to a level of experience prior to any hard and fast distinction between subjectivity and objectivity.) To repeat, illness manifests itself somatically and these manifestations guide the work of the physician. Thus, our understanding of illness requires a phenomenological approach to these somatic manifestations. Careful, nuanced descriptions of somatic phenomena, contributing to a phenomenology of illness, are critical for securing a sufficiently thick description of the relevant contexts.

But this does not make illness simply a somatic state or condition. Illness is rather an alteration in *our comportment toward the world.* It is, first and foremost, a modification of our orientation toward the everyday. The relevant phenomena – the most salient ways in which illness *shows* (or announces) itself – are in effect somatic signs, *broadly conceived:* the manifest intimates the latent, the perceptible insinuates the hidden, but this occurs in reference to what Maxine Sheets-Johnstone calls intercorporeality,[2] not only (not even primarily) in reference to the body either in isolation from others or in abstraction from its engagements with the world. That is, illness reveals itself in how a body comports itself toward other bodies as well as how a body appears other than itself (other than it ordinarily or normally appears). Most critically, it concerns the human body as a social actor in relationship to other such actors but also to the repertoire of its abilities, capacities, and susceptibilities (Merleau-Ponty). And this brings me to a *clinical* point. Our understanding of illness is inherently normative and the norms definitive of illness are, in any given culture, ones bearing upon how embodied, social selves ought to comport themselves toward one another and toward themselves. The *clinical* is that which pertains to the observation and treatment of the ill; it implies the accredited expertise of culturally recognized authorities, that is, authoritative interpreters of the somatic signs allegedly indicative of human illnesses.

I use here the term *illness* rather than *disease* not only because of the title of this colloquium. I also use the term to challenge the dualism between illness and disease so prevalent in so much of the clinical discourse regarding human maladies. In challenging this dualism, I hope also to work toward deconstructing the dichotomy of the expert third-person perspective of the clinician and the unreliable first-person perspective of the patient.[3] The primordial human perspective is, arguably, neither the first- nor the third-person perspective, but rather *the second-person perspective* (the position of being addressed by another self). I am able to think (converse with myself) and speak (converse with others) only because others have conversed with me, addressed me when I was an infant (responded to spontaneous movements and sounds as expressions, apart from anything I could have originally intended). One reason to emphasize the second-person perspective here is the way the first-person perspective is so quickly and completely identified with a subjective (rather than intersubjective and indeed intercorporeal). It is *the I in its interchangeable or dialogical relationship to the Thou* – what Peirce called *tuism* [*tu* = you or Thou, i.e., second person] – that matters here: it is the *I* as addressing or addressed by *you* or some other that is of utmost importance. This accords the first-person perspective its due but does so in such a way to underscore its indissoluble link to the second-person perspective: *you* address me and, in turn, *I* address you, in a process in which neither the *arché* nor the *telos* (neither the inaugural utterance or immanent goal) of the exchange is fixed in advance or transparent to the participants.

The relevance of these considerations to the topic at hand is that illness is, *as a clinical phenomenon* (at least, as a clinical phenomenon considered in light of an archeological approach), neither an objectively certified condition nor a subjectively felt state. It is *an intersubjectively negotiated position* and, at least by implication, a narratively constituted stance toward world and self. The narrative might be as simple as this: the doctor informed me of having cancer and, given her diagnosis and prognosis of the form of cancer I have, convinced me to accept her recommendation to undergo a particular round of onerous treatments. But my condition, even as nothing more than a condition (i.e., conceived as something less than an alteration of my comportment toward the world), is unintelligible to me *apart from the narrative,* no matter how elliptically recalled or reconstructed, of how I came to learn of this condition and also how I came to concur with the recommendations of my physician. The intelligibility of my condition depends upon my ability to relate it to antecedent affairs and exchanges, on the one hand, and intended endeavors and subjections, on the other. In brief, it assumes the shape of a story.

If illness is not only an intersubjectively but also a narratively negotiated position in the world, then the relevance of literature to the practice of medicine is fairly straightforward. Later, however, I will highlight not so much the narrative as the *dialogical* aspects of literary texts and the pertinence of these aspects to a deeper comprehension of what medical practice invariably involves. At this juncture, let me simply stress, by way of anticipation, the way *intersecting dialogues* (including here the exchanges between patient and physician as well as those at the heart of literature) tend to enrich, enhance, and deepen but also disrupt one another.

To investigate *illness in context,* paying especially close attention to the archeological, phenomenological, and clinical contexts in and through which illness attains its humanly recognizable and culturally specific shapes, requires us to contextualize our own investigations. It requires us to situate our own efforts in an explicitly *semiotic*, *hermeneutic*, and *narrative* framework. I cannot even remotely come close to accomplishing this within the confines of this essay. But let me go some distance, however small, toward this goal, attending above all to the semiotic framework in which a discussion of the signs of illness and, moreover, the pathologies of interpretation might most fruitfully be undertaken.

2. Toward a Comprehensive Theory of Our Signifying Practices

The theory of signs is rooted in our various uses of signs, in our diverse practices of everyday conversation,[4] medical diagnosis, scientific investigation, artistic innovation, and moral deliberation. These practices in all their variety and variability are primary, whereas our theoretical accounts of this vast spectrum of human practices are secondary: more simply, our uses of signs are primary, our theories of this uses are derivative. But theories are themselves forms of practice: they are historically evolved and evolving ways of striving to accomplish certain objectives (often objectives not conceivable, let alone attainable, apart from these practices). In addition, the conclusions of our theoretical practices (e.g., medical research and literary theory) are often woven into the fabric of our everyday ones.

Theories are (to repeat) forms of practice and, as such, they are modes of engagement with some identifiable region of experience. The engagement of theorists with the objects of their discourse might be complexly mediated and apparently distant, but the quality of their theorizing is ultimately dependent on the depth of their engagement (at least, on the depth of engagement made possible by this theorizing). Thus, the bearing of our theories on experience, both the domain of experience with which they are immediately preoccupied and other domains to which they might turn out to be applicable, is ultimately regulative. A theorist might however strategically treat this bearing as negligible. At various junctures, they might pay little or no attention to the specific details of the experiential regions to which their theories are, in the last analysis, responsible. On the one hand, it is necessary to defend here the *free play of the theoretical imagination.*[5] Such imagination and thus theory itself can serve experience best when it is not tied too anxiously or too narrowly to how the assertions, hypotheses, and images prompted by this play directly (or immediately) bear upon the disclosures of experience. On the other hand, it is also necessary to insist upon the *ultimate* responsibility of theorists to do the fullest justice to the actual disclosures of human experience. The play of imagination and our fidelity to experience are, hence, equally important in this connection.

The self-controlled use of signs depends upon a self-critical awareness of their operation, influence, and indeed simply their presence. In turn, self-criticism depends on self-consciousness, on becoming aware more explicitly and focally of what we are doing, of how we are using signs in this or that context. In brief, self-control depends on self-criticism and, in turn, self-criticism depends on self-consciousness. But the self-consciousness so necessary for evaluating and altering our use of signs is always akin to the self-consciousness so inimical to the graceful performance of even the most solidly consolidated habits (or habitual actions). Think here of being so self-conscious in walking across a stage that one stumbles or, at best, moves in an exceedingly awkward and unnatural manner; or think of being so self-conscious in a conversation that one stutters, even though one virtually never experiences such difficulty in speaking. Self-consciousness can certainly undermine the fluid or graceful performances (or enactments) of unreflective agents. But, unreflective agency can, in turn, rest upon systematic blindness to a large number of potentially salient elements in a practical situation (a context in which an agent, ordinarily in concert with other, is called upon to act – e.g., to greet a patient, to suggest a course of treatment, or to issue a directive to a co-worker). The fluency of the callous or inconsiderate actor should be checked; a halting self-consciousness here is desirable.

'The most important moment in the history of a sign or a set [system] of signs is,' according to David Savan, 'the point at which deliberate critical appraisal of the norms themselves [the norms governing the use of this sign or system] begins.' He immediately adds: 'It is at this point that thought comes of age and that mature science is born'.[6] This is not only the point at which science attains maturity; it is also one at which signifying practices quite distinct from the idealized form of experimental investigation (i.e., from the paradigm of *science* it it's distinctively modern form) reach a *critical* phase in their ongoing evolution. Medicine and literature clearly illustrate this point. In mostly different ways, both are fields in which the operative and indeed constitutive norms and ideals defining a field of activity (e.g., the practice of dealing with the ill or that of narrating the complex intersection of imagined lives) are, time and again, made explicit. Beyond this, these norms and ideals are themselves made the objects of 'deliberate critical appraisal'. In a concrete, practical way, an interrogation of the meanings of illness and its most appropriate treatments are integral to the practice of medicine, just as a questioning of the nature of (say) narration and its diverse forms are integral to the practices of storytellers. Medicine and literature take a *critical* turn when such self-interrogation becomes a pervasive, transformative, and indeed constitutive aspect of these practices (medical doctors *are* those preoccupied with the question of the meaning of illness, just as literary artists are those preoccupied with the forms, possibilities, and effects of, say, narrative). This is a point especially worth of our consideration, since it involves an ordinarily unmarked affinity between medicine and literature.

3. Literature *and* Medicine

Though in very different ways, medicine and literature bear upon 'the deliberate critical appraisals of the norms' inherent in – indeed, partly constitutive of – one of more forms of human practice. *Medicine* does so primarily by critically appraising it's most basic norm – that of health – but also the criteria by which the ascription of health and, conversely, that of illness are experimentally warranted. In contrast, *literature* serves this task principally in a twofold way – first, by bringing into focus the operative norms in a given culture and, second, by adopting an experimental attitude toward the inherent norms of literary production itself (by trying out, for example, new modes of narration, ones wherein the traditional norms of narrative discourse are exposed in all their conventionality). Much more can and, for that matter, should be said about how medicine and literature exemplify the tendency of a signifying practice to evolve to the point where 'the deliberate critical appraisal of norms' become integral to the practice itself. Questions of the meaning of health and healing come to be, time and again, focal concerns of the medical profession, just as questions concerning the meaning of literature as a cultural practice are hardly ever extrinsic to the crafting of some literary texts in virtually every epoch in which there is any evidence of literary production. Though much more should be said about this and related topics, it is sufficient, for the purpose at hand, simply to note that these signifying practices bear in complex ways upon the critical assessment of various norms, most immediately norms constitutive of these practices themselves but ultimately a wide range of (apparently) extrinsic norms, i.e., norms embodied in other signifying practices.

While much is controversial about both medicine and especially literature, this much seems beyond dispute. Two of our most important signifying practices are the *medical* deployment of signs for purposes of diagnosis and prognosis[7] as well as the *artistic* deployment of linguistic signs for any number of purposes.[8] 'Literature is,' according to Jonathan Culler, 'the most interesting case of semiosis for a variety of reasons.' One important reason is that literature 'forces one to face the problem of the indeterminacy of meaning, which is a central if paradoxical property of semiotic systems'.[9]

Arguably, medicine is an equally interesting case of semiosis, principally for the reason that the family of practices subsumed under this heading is predicated on the recognition of the problem of the indeterminacy of meaning, but nonetheless committed to the practical delimitation of the polysemous signs (and thus indeterminate meanings) of its most basic terms (e.g., illness, disease, cure, health, and wellness).

The development of medical *practice* is accordingly one with the development of a particular enhancement of semiotic competency, one with the evolution of the identification, interpretation, and appraisal of the signs of illness. The *practice of medicine* provides valuable material for a comprehensive articulation of the *theory of signs*. In his efforts to craft a truly encompassing theory of signs, C. S. Peirce (1834-1914) attends to the symptom as a sign of illness and, moreover, categorizes it as a legisign: 'The symptom itself is a legisign, a general type of a definite character.' The actual occurrence in any particular case is, in contrast, a sinsign.[10] The work of Eugen Baer and others has demonstrated in detail how much Peirce's finely drawn distinctions and even forbiddingly technical terms help to illuminate the practice of medicine. It also helps to offer a systematic account of our accredited practices of diagnosing, monitoring, and curing illnesses. But, on this occasion, pathological modes of interpreting signs (including the somatic signs of human illness) deserves at least as much consideration as our accredited forms of interpreting them.

4. Crisscrossing Dialogues: Experience, Literature, & Medicine

Part of the value of literature in reference to enhancing our understanding of illness pertains directly to issues of re-contextualization and, more generally, contextualization. One of the ways in which literature enhances this understanding is by vividly portraying 'the intimacies of the direct contacts and intercourses of life,' precisely at those moments or phases in which life as the result of illness withdraws within itself. Illness is not simply a somatic state but a worldly orientation: it is a quality of our comportment toward 'the world of things and persons' such that our ordinary modes of comportment (or engagement) are reduced in some appreciable and *felt* degree – or *if* these modes of comportment *are* sustained, they are so with far greater effort and pain than is normally the case.

Another way in which literature enhances our comprehension of illness is by bringing into focus the cultural contexts and, inherent in such complex inheritances, the conflicting interpretations and indeed rival authorities concerning the nature, causes, and forms of illness.

Yet another way in which literature can deepen our understanding of illness is by (in effect) exhibiting some facet of the very structure of experience, of making available for reflection – for interpretation and appraisal – some aspect of the *dialogue between self and world,* some feature of the ongoing exchange between symbol-using animals such as human beings and a symbol-generating matrix such as the world of our experience (a world in no slight measure intelligible in diverse ways, no matter how opaque and enigmatic in other respects).

Experience as a dialogue between self and world is profoundly enhanced by literature as itself a dialogue between author and a number of other factors (not the least of all, natural languages, literary traditions, cultural norms, and rival discourses), also by literature as a dialogue between reader and text.

We certainly might be surprised along with Virginia Woolf that 'illness has not taken its place with love and battle and jealousy among the prime themes of literature'.[11] But the bearing of literature on the theme of illness has been arguably far greater than Woolf realized. Moreover, the literature written since 1930, the year when her 'On Being Ill' was published has perhaps made more of this theme than literature before this time.

Woolf's own illnesses and indeed suicide, no less than her writings, aid us in imagining why illness deserves to take its place, among the themes of literature, alongside 'love and battle and jealousy'. For what they reveal is nothing less than this. The dialogue of self and world is not infrequently broken off, insofar as this is possible, in various ways, not least of all by the more or less uncontrollable withdrawal of the self from the world, i.e., of the self into itself (the sort of withdrawal identifiable with illness). The fate of illness can invite or even enforce reflection on the meaning of health. Such reflection can turn critical attention away from the signs of illness and toward the illnesses of signs, the undetected symptoms of a relentless drive to make determinate sense of especially the recurrent, perceptible forms so crucial for rendering our experience intelligible. Here also Woolf is insightful. She observes:

> In illness words seem to possess a mystic quality. We grasp what is beyond their surface meaning, gather instinctively this, that, and the other – a sound, a colour, [a fragrance], here a stress, there a pause – which the poet, knowing words to be meagre in comparison with ideas, has strewn about his page to evoke, when collected, a state of mind which neither words can express nor the reason explain. Incomprehensibility has an enormous power over us in illness, more legitimately perhaps than the upright [or healthy] will allow. In health meaning has encroached upon sound [has so thoroughly and immediately encroached upon sound that its textures, timbre, rhythms are all but

> unheard]. Our intelligence domineers over our senses. But in illness, with the police off duty, we creep beneath some obscure poem by Mallarmé or Donne, some phrase in Latin or Greek, and the words give out their scent and distil their flavour, and then, if at last we grasp the meaning, it is all the richer for having come to us sensually first, by way of the palate or the nostrils, like some queer odour. Foreigners, to whom the tongue is strange, have us at a disadvantage. The Chinese must know the sound of *Anthony and Cleopatra* better than we do.[12]

But the 'mystic quality' attaching to words and other signs as a result of illness might be even more radical than Woolf appears to allow in this passage. The illness of inherent in our irrepressible and often desperate reliance on signs – the illness of signs themselves – is inseparable from the effective annihilation of any vivid sense of, lively feel for, qualitative immediacy, quite apart from the contribution of such immediacy to the conveyance of meaning. Illness can release us from the imperative to make sense of the sights and sights, smells and twinges, to which the body (as much as death) is heir. In illness, words and other signs can 'give out their scent and distil their flavour' for their own sake and, thereby, cease to be words and signs. The value of illness can be a release from the demands of significance, because it can provide an immersion in the play of sense, a giving of the self to rapturous absorption in qualitative immediacy. If this occurs, illness provides a lesson for understanding vitality and health. But, *in itself,* the meaning of illness resides not so much in any lessons it might provide for understanding vitality or health or anything else, as it resides in exposing the extent to which we are afflicted by the illness of meaning, the inability to be enlivened by the sheer qualitative immediacy of felt experience. To use Peirce's categories, the sense of secondness so predominant in the experience of illness – the sense of simply *not* feeling well, of being *other than* our ordinary selves, of *not* having the energy or capacity to do what our healthy selves can so readily and unreflectively accomplish – [to repeat, the sense of secondness so predominant in the experience of illness] should be permitted to eclipse the sense of firstness (the quality of what Woolf calls mysticism) inherent in illness.

The dialogue of self and world is, thus, one in which our qualisigns (those qualities we have pressed into the service of signification) might dissolve into qualities having no role or importance other than their immediately felt being here and now. Incomprehensibility has indeed 'an enormous power over us in illness,' an even greater power than Woolf seems to acknowledge. An anxious solicitude regarding significance is suspended, replaced by an unapologetic embrace of the sheer incomprehensibility of the felt qualities of lived experience. The qualities of our experience require no justification or warrant other than their appearance.

The dialogue of self and world is broadened and deepened by the engagement of the self with literature. For virtually everyone reading this essay, the dialogue between reader and text is inseparable from *this* engagement: the dialogue of self and world *is* in no small measure the engagement of self with literature. But, *on falling ill,* our comportment toward the world is altered (or if our characteristic comportment toward the world is even approximately maintained, it is only by a greater effort and at greater pain than is normally the case). On being ill, however, our comportment toward the world as a sphere of significance can be radically transformed. In light of such transformations, it becomes no less imperative to note the degree to which the demand for meaning can itself be a sign of illness than the various pathological forms of interpretation. Being ill, precisely because it involves being *other than* our ordinary selves, allows for the immediacies of experience *to be themselves,* simply what they are in themselves, apart from all else (in particular, apart from their role in conveying meaning). In other words, being ill, because of its secondness, its otherness from normalcy, allows for firstness, not just the firstness of being ill but the firstness of all else.

Woolf suggests that, without the help of the poets, 'we can but trifle'.[13] With the visions provided by them, we are afforded the possibility 'to live and live till we have lived out those embryo lives which attend about us in early youth until 'I' suppressed them'.[14] Illness can conspire with poetry (or literature) to suppress the suppressing 'I,' to undermine not only the narrowing drive for meaning but also the suffocating sovereignty of the self. To be deprived of our ordinary self can be as much (if not more) an opportunity as a deprivation: it can be an opportunity to return to that time when our own largely unformed lives contained within themselves those 'embryo lives' all too soon suppressed by a sovereign self.

5. Conclusion

The individuals who arise from a sick bed, especially if they have not only lost themselves in the utterly irresponsible play of felt qualities but also if they have found themselves back with the unrealized selves of their own distant pasts (or simply found themselves amid the hitherto unimagined selves suggested from unimaginably diverse sources), might be quite different selves than those who took to bed in the first place.

Interpreting the signs of illness has the potential to expose our commitment to intelligibility and thus interpretation as itself symptomatic of a deficiency, if not truly an illness. *Contextualizing* our manner of interpreting such signs – *first*, in terms of the context of immediate personal experience, *second*, in terms of relevant cultural contexts, and, finally, in terms of a comprehensive understanding of the structure or human experience – provides us with a criterion by which to determine the possibly pathological character of our various hermeneutic strategies.

The theory of signs is rooted in our practices of using signs in various contexts for various purposes. The fuller justice such a theory does to the widest array of such practices, the more comprehensive and adequate is such a theory. Moreover, the theory of signs is itself a practice that has evolved from practices of a less formally self-conscious and self-critical character. The evolution of this theory depends, above all else, on the complex interplay between two dynamic factors – the free play of the theoretical imagination and a fidelity to the disclosures of experience.

Illness as well as literature can contribute to both of these factors. Both do so not least of all by exposing the unsuspected limitations and distortions inherent in our habitual or customary frames of meaning. They expose these limitations and distortions by suggesting alternative frames, rival schemes, of intelligibility. The movement back and forth from wider to narrower spheres of significance is a mark of intellectual vitality and health, whereas the inability to move from more restricted to more encompassing contexts – and back again – is a symptom of intellectual illness. Even more radically, illness and literature can expose the dulling or deadening of sensibility that results from a tyrannical preoccupation with significance, a stultifying fixation on intelligibility. This is one of the most important respects in which both are potentially liberating. To be relieved of the demand to make sense of our experience in the inherited terms of even our most adequate discourses is frequently welcome and even exhilarating. But, to be relieved of the demand to make sense at all – simply *to be* and to be without any felt need for justification or explanation – is to enter that foreign country[15] in which, paradoxically, we frequently feel most intimately at home. Illness thus can be a homecoming to a foreign country as well as a number of other paradoxical, fateful positions into which the frailties of our bodies and the complicities of our psyches thrust us.

The most pathological frameworks of interpretation are, accordingly, precisely those that occlude the *fateful paradoxes of illness* in their irreducibly paradoxical and uniquely fateful character. From a semiotic and hermeneutic perspective, no signs of illness are more troubling than those indicating the loss of self, not least of all the self as co-narrator of the course of that self's experience. Such signs ineluctably prefigure death. But the experience of the self, *palpably* confronted with the loss of the everyday world along with that of its self, can be an intense, exhilarating, and even liberating experience. This and other paradoxes pertaining to illness are, I propose, among the phenomena most worthy of our deliberate critical appraisal. The intersecting of medicine and literature does not merely make such appraisal possible. It makes such consideration necessary, even urgent.

Notes

[1] W Nöth, *Handbook of Semiotics*, Indiana University Press, Bloomington IN, 1990.

[2] M Sheets-Johnstone, *Roots of Power: Animate Form and Gendered Bodies*, Open Court, La Salle, IL, 1994, pp. 34, 57-59, 110.

[3] DB Morris, *Illness and Culture in the Postmodern Age*, University of California Press, Berkeley, 1998, p. 37.

[4] In MS 283, C. S. Peirce asserts, the more perfectly anything fulfills its function as a sign, 'the less effect it has upon that quasi-mind [that upon which it exerts its influence] than that of determining it [the quasi-mind] as if the object itself had acted upon it. Thus, after an ordinary conversation, a wonderfully perfect kind of sign functioning, one knows what information or suggestion has been conveyed, but will be utterly unable to say in what words it was conveyed, and often will think it was conveyed in words, when in fact it was only conveyed in tones or in facial expressions' (EP 2, 391),

[5] Peirce claims, 'there is, after all, nothing but imagination that can ever supply him [the scientist] an inkling of the truth' (CP 1.46). After the 'passion to learn' – the drive to discover what is not yet known – 'there is no quality so indispensable to the successful prosecution of science as imagination' (CP 1. 47).

[6] D Savan, *An Introduction to C. S. Peirce's Full System of Semiotic*, Toronto Semiotic Circle, Toronto, 1987-88, p. 63; cf. Colapietro.

[7] Nöth.

[8] In *Art as Experience,* Dewey suggests: 'Ultimately there are but two philosophies. One of them accepts life and [thus embraces] experience in all its uncertainty, mystery, doubt, and half-knowledge and turns that experience upon itself to deepen and intensify its own qualities – to imagination and art. This is the philosophy of Shakespeare and Keats' *(LW* 10, 41). The process of *turning experience upon itself* for the sake of

deepening and intensifying its own inherent qualities, in both their qualitative immediacy and indeliminable suggestiveness (both the textures of feeling and the intimations of intelligibility), seems to be one of the most distinctive functions of artworks, especially from the modern epoch to the present. Such a function can thus be a self-consciously espoused purpose on the part of the artist: it guides – informs and animates – the artistic deployment of signs.

[9] J Culler, 'In Defense of Overinterpretation' in *Interpretation and Overinterpretation*, S Collini (ed), 1981, p. 35.

[10] CS Peirce, *Collected Papers of Charles Sanders Peirce,* volume 8, A Burks (ed), Belknap Press at Harvard University Press, Cambridge, MA, 1958, p. 335.

[11] V Woolf, 'On Being Ill' in *Collected Essays,* volume 4, The Hogarth Press, London, 1967, (1930), p. 193.

[12] ibid., p. 200.

[13] ibid., p. 199.

[14] ibid., p. 199.

[15] Sontag.

Bibliography

Barthes, R., 'Sémiologie et médicine'. *Les sciences de la folie,* Bastide, R. (ed), 1972.

Cassell, E.J., 'Illness & Disease'. *Hastings Center Report* 6, no. 2, 1976.

Chekhov, A., *Ward No. 6 & Other Stories*. Translated by Constance Garnett, Barnes & Noble Classics, NY, 2003.

Colapietro, V., 'Natural processes and historical practices: Towards a postmodern cosmology of human semiosis'. *Semiotica*, 119-1/2, 1998.

Colapietro, V., 'Peirce the contrite fallibilist, convinced pragmaticist, and critical commonsensist' in *Semiotica* 111-1/2, 1996.

Collini, S. (ed), *Interpretation and Overinterpretation*. Cambridge University Press, Cambridge, 1992.

Culler, J., 'In Defense of Overinterpretation' in *Interpretation and Overinterpretation*. Stefan Collini (ed), 1992.

Culler, J., *The Pursuit of Signs: Semiotics, Literature, & Deconstruction*. Cornell University Press, Ithaca, NY, 1981.

Dewey, J., 'The Unity of the Human Bering' in *Later Works of John Dewey*. Volume 13, JA Boydston (ed), SIU Press, Carbondale, IL, 1991. [Originally, an address to the American College of Physicians, St. Louis, MO, 21 April 1937].

Dewey, J., *Art as Experience. Later Works of John Dewey*. Volume 10, J A Boydston (ed), SIU Press, Carbondale, IL, 1989 (1934).

Dewey, J., 'Context and Thought'. *Later Works of John Dewey*. Volume 6, J A Boydston (ed), SIU Press, Carbondale, IL, 1931.

Dewey, J., *The Quest for Certainty. Later Works of John Dewey*. Volume 4, J A Boydston (ed), SIU Press, Carbondale, IL, 1988 (1929).

Eco, U., 'Overinterpreting Texts'. *Interpretation and Overinterpretation*. S Collini (ed), 1992.

Fisch, M.H., *Peirce, Semeiotic, and Pragmatism*. K L Ketner and C J W Kloesel (eds), Indiana University Press, Bloomington, IN, 1986.

Fulford, K.W.M., *Moral Theory & Practice*. Cambridge University Press, Cambridge, 1989.

Gerhardt, U., *Ideas About Illness: An Intellectual & Political History of Medical Sociology*. NYU Press, NY, 1989.

Hudson, R.P., 'Concepts of Disease in the West'. *The Cambridge World History of Disease*. Kiple, K.P. (ed), Cambridge University Press, NY, 1993.

Leder, D., *The Absent Body*. University of Chicago Press, Chicago, 1990.

Morris, D.B., *Illness and Culture in the Postmodern Age*. University of California Press, Berkeley, 2000.

Nöth, W., *Handbook of Semiotics*. Indiana University Press, Bloomington, IN, 1990.

Olds, S., *The Father*. Knopf, NY, 1992.

Peirce, C.S. *The Essential Peirce: Selected Philosophical Writings*. Volume 2 (1893-1913), Peirce Edition Project (ed), Indiana University Press, Bloomington, IN, 1992.

Peirce, C.S., *Collected Papers of Charles Sanders Peirce*. Volume 8, A Burks (ed), Belknap Press at Harvard University Press, Cambridge, MA, 1958.

Peschel, E.R. (ed.), *Medicine and Literature*. Neale Watson Academic Publications, Inc., NY, 1980.

Rorty, R., 'Objectivity, Relativism, & Truth'. *Philosophical Papers,* volume 1. Cambridge University Press, Cambridge, 1991.

Sachs, O., *An Anthropologist on Mars: Seven paradoxical Tales*. Knopf, NY, 1995.

Savan, D., *An Introduction to C. S. Peirce's Full System of Semeiotic*. Toronto Semiotic Circle, Toronto, 1987-88.

Schatzki, T.R., Karin K.C. and Eike von Savigny (eds), *The Practice Turn in Contemporary Theory*. Routledge, London, 2001.

Sheets-Johnstone, M., *Roots of Power: Animate Form and Gendered Bodies*. Open Court, La Salle, IL, 1994.

Short, T.L., 'Peirce's Theory of Signs'. *Cambridge Companion to Peirce*, C Misak (ed)., 2004.

Smith, J.E., 'Philosophical Interpretation and the religious Dimension of Experience'. *Logos,* 2, 1981.

Sontag, S., *Illness as Metaphor & AIDS & Its Metaphors*. Picador, NY, 2001.

Staiano, K.V., *Interpreting Signs of Illness: A Case Study in Medical Semiotics*. Mouton de Gruyter, Berlin,1986.

Woolf, V., 'On Being Ill'. *Collected Essays,* volume 4, The Hogarth Press, London, 1967 (1930).

II - PHENOMENOLOGY

From *The Day I Wasn't There*

Hélène Cixous

Key Words: Down's syndrome; family history; women's inner landscape.

*****

I never think of my son the dead, I thought toward my cat who was smiling at me with her minimissimal overwhelming smile, while she watched me think on her, bearing the unspeakable mess of my mental images with the compassion that comes to her aid with my convulsions. I never think of my son the dead and that is not an exaggeration for even when he comes to mind it is not I who think of him, it is he who steals with his congenital modesty into a far corner of the room where he ends up melting away without my having made a move in his direction. He is not one to make a fuss. And even at this moment when my son the dead was the direct object of my thoughts, indirectness reigned and I did not try to curtail it. My cat leapt delicately at my nose so as to join her soul to mine in this visibly gloomy meditation. While I, I didn't budge toward my son the dead. And his nose—have I ever licked or caressed it? I could say that it's all the fault of the verb *to think*; it is because of the way it is constructed, its manner of taking an indirect object, by which it means to signify its circuitousness and precaution to us, it is a verb that prowls, a dreamy sort of action. It is a roundabout process. One must go toward the dead son and that takes time in my case it is going to take up to decades. In the old days perhaps I thought of my son directly but I do not think to remember that. Or maybe it's linked to the actualization of the verb *to think*, to the intransitiveness of its construction.

But what I see rather is that when it comes to my son I have always been indirect and vice versa, we were fated. Fate is what we have in common. Whereas *ponder* in its etymological sense, 'to weigh,' is transitive. But that's just it *I was never able to weigh my son*, I could not weigh him, without being caught up and overcome by an invincible terror, with the result that after a few months three or four I believe I'd given up weighing him, because weighing him for me it was as if each time I was sentenced anew, weighing him was to hear the pitiless word of the scales all over again why bother consulting them, they prophesied to me in vain, perhaps that's when I began weighing him indirectly and without noticing it became perpetual. When he reached four and a half kilos, exhausted, which I don't say to excuse myself, and besides terrorized rather than worn out, I handed him over to my mother. In order to set between us a space for thought. I gave him to my mother to weigh, without consciously knowing that I was giving my mother the whole child including the final act, exit, and epilogue.

Only to my cat, keeper of my sorrows and sentences which for me in the inside of me remain secret, can I recall this: For I do nothing else: A brief and frail evocation not much more than a flame, that is all that glimmers and remains of the vast, grave lost continent of my son the dead. Whoever has never contemplated such a flame, *the yartseit candle*, the one they would light in my family one week in February, does not know the wretched glimmer of mourning, and has never seen with his own eyes the cruel, very cruel miserly misfortune represented with a dreadful meticulousness in this very poor, very pitiful icon. One sticks a wick in a kitchen glass formerly filled with mustard filled with oil and set next to a photo of the deceased, in the form of a bad enlargement of an identity photo. I saw death in a photo: I saw death. Everything is blurred, cut, abandoned. The head is just a small portion of the body. No body. The impotence of the regretful dead. It's him, for sure. The dead's photo. The eternal flame tarnished by oil, coated alive in a film of grime. The scene is faithful in every detail to the fate of the dead. At the end of his rope, at the end of the light, at the end of looking, at the end of memory. You can tell in the distance he weighs nothing.

And so, on this First of May, without meaning to, someone had lit for me the brief, sad beam of mourning that signals the dishonoring of the dead.

It came from the family papers, the unexpected gleam. It was because I'd made a photocopy of the irreparable documents destined long since to destruction and dispersion. Compared with my grandmother's and my mother's sturdy German documents which survived the century's brutal moves, these were destined to dislocation from the very day they were fabricated. In vain does one tape the pages back into the City of Algiers's official certificates of birth and death, nothing stops the ungluing. The leaves suffered no attempt at reassembly. As I was on the point of confiding the tattered bundle to my son the wind, I had the idea of keeping some trace of a thing in its agony. And presto, up it came, good as new, a neat and tidy ghost considerably stronger than the real thing. Photocopied. As a result of this undertaking that which had been falling apart found itself together again, just like that: It told an unexpectedly modern tale, in which events make a mockery of chronological order, hence reading from west to east, I divorced on the left before bringing my daughter into the world on the right, and on the following page I suddenly saw and for the first time ever in living memory my two sons side by side preceded and thus heralded by the death sentence of my son declared dead before he was born officially.

My two sons before me together, I'd never experienced that. Side by side my two sons with death at their side, that's how they came to me. I never thought of it I thought, I never put two and two together that way, to see them lying next to one another under my eyes now, two brothers gazing up at their mother, and that happened all at once and it happened in the furthest reach of my being, it raced along my nerves with the speed of lightning, it coursed through my body like the annunciation of pregnancy, I felt the first contraction, first sign, the same as the desire for love and right away your breasts hurt and immediately came the flood of tears, the same for the shock of love when at the moment we embrace one another with the hardness of those whom the imminence of loss galvanizes we keep check on our soul abrim with thoughts which however we do not locate: We merely escape the abyss which remains agape.

Surprised, I wept. And I don't know why. Maternity rendered, maternity lost. It was for lack of thought and the fault of words

One of my sons is dead
The other is alive
How to think that
One of my sons is still alive
The other is dead
One of my sons is still dead
The other is very much alive
How to think that

My son the one who is dead, my former son my son who is no longer my son. And the one I call my son is my son the living. The other is outside, he was there for so long that I never think of him to his face.

My cat weighs four and a half kilos. I carry her around on my shoulder making sure she is holding on tight, I sing songs to her eyes.

How to ponder the weight the place the replacement the tenacity of the speechless who ask for nothing, who glimmer in a corner of your heart? How to answer the question: How many children did you have, without long, slow reflection, going back over youths and old ages, without interrogating each word of this question which interrogates me in every part of my being as if I could count up and arrive at the sum of what is still more child than child what is less child than child? You had children? Yes yes yes, how many? Oh, that! it depends. Since the apparition of my son the lamb with his webbed hands, there is an Impossibility, since the unheralded arrival of my son the Impossible, I can't say how many without the words *how many* coming undone, the child too, undone, fended off and defended and de-fended from within, how many children? That is why the day of the apparition, head turned toward the square window at which press a herd of creatures their faces a little fishlike who gaze at me through the square of glass, mouthing O, I hesitate to string together a proper sentence, with a to have and a to be in it. It's as if at the moment I was trying to answer for myself, an abrupt sensation of something missing from my mouth, and on my lap, there's a tooth. Just before I opened it, my mouth, there were thirty-two of them and at the moment I still have thirty-two of which one is no longer within but on my lap. It is small, pearly, pointy, with a black spot at the root and carved like a cat's tooth. It's my tooth which was my tooth and is no longer my tooth. I examine it.

That is what came to happen to me in the Sainte-Foy maternity home. I see the scene as if I myself were outside pressed against the windowpane my nose squashed against the glass, my mouth round with curiosity. I see it. She, that's me that day who just got tipped out of myself and no way to climb back into the house of me from which I have fallen. Time pivots and falls. There is no more past. The future not yet. What remains is a hesitation of ill-attached ill-detached present hanging over the two beds the big one and the little one. Outside the fish swim round the aquarium.

She can't get over it. She lingers in a bizarre hour, adrift, between two hours. She has just given birth, for one thing. For another, what has happened it's that the one who has just been born, he hasn't quite yet arrived anywhere, he is not in his place, he wriggles weakly still in the wings, offstage as if detained by a tremendous uncertainty, as if timid. As for her she doesn't move, she waits. For the place. She doesn't think: What a surprise this child, this child which doesn't seem to be hers, who differs, who doesn't look like, this fish gasping as if it needed to go back in the water, one expects a surprise but instead of the expected surprise it's an entirely different one, O mysterious power of the new arrival who upsets the millions of expectations of millenniums of images, O eternally astonishing natural phenomenon forever never seen before. And this one here, he's the champion. He evades her absolutely, she doesn't remember him at all. She doesn't conceive of him. She has come to a stop. Where? At the stop.

I see the woman do silent battle with the child, this is in one of those worlds where on the threshold a spell is cast over whoever strays or ventures in, where the laws of metamorphosis reign, where one never knows who pursues whom for dozens of light-years, where one cannot not hunt as one breathes. I see the woman and child beasts, held alive in the burning frost of a face-to-face the way two cats caught in the last two meters of a kingdom stand still for hours guarding the last two meters with the patient tenacity of gods measuring out between them their last chance at immortality.

The way two heroes advance toward the final instant slowly sharing the taste of each inch of white sand, which is what they have in common, this morsel of earthly fabric which kisses their feet, they do not run they revel together in what unites them in a loving hostility, this space which is not going to last, which they are going to cut, unequally, this solemn diminution.

They stare at one another, distractedly, that's what's strange.

The woman glances out of the corner of her eye at the face of the one who has just arrived, oblique. Then she jerks her head away as if fearing some danger, darts a glance in the direction of the window on the other side of which the bizarre spectators are pressed together, then brings all her power of inquiry to bear on the face of the child. On his face is an absence. Something unfocused maybe. A kind of veil. You couldn't say she dotes on him. She bends an ear. She tries to make out what the sentences are whispering to her, rushing past like sighs.

It's that there is something in the back of her mind that she can't quite grasp yet she feels a form devoid of strength flit by or on the contrary a form monstrously strong in its weakness. The vague child. At the pane the crowd presses in.

A sentence says: 'What has just happened' and she hears the strangeness of this *what*.

What has happened is that the child in the cradle has not arrived yet, at least he hasn't been informed. He believes he is drifting, he hasn't yet landed. 'What has come to pass.' How to describe it, how to describe, this to come which has already come and which is still on the way, which hasn't finished, which isn't finished, which doesn't commence, which is all mixed up. Because if *this* has happened, it has happened but if it is still coming it's that *this* hasn't happened, which is what renders the child still intangible though in the cradle. Morphologically it's a present, but curved, melting, receding. Missing. The child has arrived, incorrect.

The woman's heart beats slowly. The child's heart beats excessively fast. This isn't it. This is not where it is. *This* is not there.

All of a sudden she thinks something crazy: He isn't horn. Does it exist, to be born without being born yet? To be almost? Almost.

On the eve of the day she gave birth she was reading *The Idiot*. Reality is a fabulous book in which everything happens when one least expects it. Everything that has never existed explodes into being from one page to the next. Fantastic plot. Chapter 7. I'm a prince. Flight. Enter the monster. Take me back home. It would have been better to nip me in the bud. A trifle. Better yet: to nip me before the bud. To have only a few months to live is this living? What is the length of that we call life? Sunrise, and the other world. One doesn't understand a thing. Being nothing, I still want. One can't not love. One doesn't know what it means to love. I see the woman bending over herself. What she calls love beats very slowly. Then suddenly excessively fast. Then very slowly.

Now she takes sides, the side of the child. The side of the vague.

She calls him.

She puts her hope in the name. She is going to catch the slippery little fish in the net of names she casts over him. Then he will turn into a little boy which is what he has not yet managed to be. She will trap him in the net of very old, strong, safe, faithful names, her secret and sacred names, and she will pull him gently out of the invisible water he has drawn around himself up to his chest.

First she calls him Adam; second she calls him George the name of her dead father who had been waiting for years to be called back among the living. Third she calls him Lev for the complicated, inexplicable Prince.

For the fourth she stops, for already she has mustered an entire army around the little boy.

She calls him.

The names are good for him. Their infinitesimal wings flutter in his ears. She has the feeling the baby is sending her tiny sounds of names soft to her ears. It's that now he's called. Now Adam, now George, now Lev. It's good for him to have such strong names, it's a whole story surrounding him, stretching far back, now he is told, he has hardly not been out his cradle she lifts him up, now he has a character, the wind blows, a diluvian storm slams into the building the weird bunch of creatures in O is swept away, firmly she holds the head of her son which is so ponderous. It is in danger of falling off, it's the neck which is awfully flexible she rocks him in her arms.

What strikes her is the lack of meanness on the extraordinarily peaceful face. It makes no sense. A mad confidence is manifest. Next to the face of her son all the newborn faces project a sour little something, a little line of defense, a scribble, a grimace. He is smooth, abstract. As if he hadn't risen. Pale, as if he hadn't finished baking.

A Nose Newborn?

Or maybe *the nose is the question*, a new noseborn in the family, which for noses always had the idea of a fin or a prehistoric flipper standing like a monolith in the middle of a delicate and well-trimmed field. See the photos of my father, with a rudder plumb in the middle.

Noticing this one-of-a-kind nose, without ancestor, without length, without idea, she feels it holds the key to the strangeness: 'What has been born to me, as if it had acceded to the objurgations of generations of my family up in arms one after another against the old nose,' she thought audacious and troubled, 'can it be a sort of non-Jew?' The blond hair the paleness as well, a son come from elsewhere, curtailed.

'I didn't want that,' she murmured to the strict and taciturn presence of her father. And yet. 'It's the rest of the family, who wanted it. Who can fathom the mysteries of creation? All of us in the family we fought over the blue blue eyes of Omi my grandmother and finally it's a great grandnephew in Australia who got them, Mendel's laws say one thing, people do something else, one doesn't give orders to the unconscious, God is an active volcano, species are reduced to ashes, new features arise, new words, new diseases, new planets, new princes, new misfortunes.'

My nose and I we have a vital relationship, a fated relationship, to which I can compare no other relation unless it is the relation with my inseparable lover. Every part of me is in keeping with this exterior and interior element of my being, everything is determined by it, for it is the only element or the only part of my vital whole which I have considered parting with. I was tempted to do it and finally after more than a year of temptation I gave up the idea of dissociating myself from it. On the subject of my nose I served the better part of my apprenticeship to good and evil, to loyalty and treason, to baseness and courage, to the mortal illness of the soul and solitude, to the lack of imagination and autoimmunity, to the proximity of the destruction of the interior treasure, and to self-hate, to the fragility of the sense of right choice and the power of attraction of the mortal enemy, to the astonishing facility with which we come to terms with those who wish us ill and whom we go out of our way to help, to the scorn we do not hesitate to inspire in ourselves, to the childish naïveté that lets us wade into shit and poison ourselves, to the complacency with which we give ourselves over to the usurpation of our own beauty. I stop.

'Get a nose job,' said my matter-of-fact mother when I arrived at the age of puberty, for it seems that this is when one has one's definitive nose. And I nearly. And I failed. I had just turned fourteen and I translated my nose into a thing for cutting, a thing of shame, a flag of ugliness flying over my countryside, into something disgusting to be got rid of. Then for a few years I didn't stop nearlying now on one side now on the other. Tugged this way and that between my father underground with his big nose and my matter-of-fact mother, for whom a nose is just a nose. Years of internal strife, wars, accusations, and denials that I never stopped bringing against myself in one way or in the other.

Finally I spared my nose that I really should have liked to cut off, but I didn't dare, for a cut nose doesn't ever grow back again, I learned that from Aeschylus.

Nose cut, terminated, once blood is spilled in the dust it doesn't rise in the veins again, that nose there, my inheritance, my father, I don't want to part with it, my father's ghost haunted me and spoke not a word, which condemned me to a difficult liberty.

I was afraid of cutting myself off from my father.

Not that my mother'd got it wrong. For two or three years I never went out with my nose naked, I went through the streets of Algiers with my nose under the fingers of my left hand as if I were trying not to sneeze, I kept it out of sight.

Lots of the things I think or act go back to my nose. Mostly negative.

Nor can one simply say that I didn't cut it off. During my Nez Caché period it was as if I cut it off to go out and stuck it back when I returned to my room. I put back the cut and the join each in turn, and I couldn't see where the crisis would end.

It was pure luck that I still had my nose when I left Algeria. Today we are reconciled, one thing is forgiven, but nothing is forgotten. It's peace head on but not in profile.

—It's all Hitler's fault, says Aunt Eri my mother's sister. We do whatever he wants without meaning to.—But me when I was over there I didn't know Hitler and you didn't either says my mother.—It's that there wasn't any television, we'd never seen Hitler, says my aunt, one didn't see him.—But me when I came to visit Omi in 1933 says my mother, my uncle, and all the gentlemen of the consistory, they were in jail, 'for their own protection.' But nobody'd seen Hitler. There was always a *gesunder Antisemitismus* as they used to say, says my aunt, but one got along very well with this *Antisemitismus*. Only one time I had a problem because I had my nose done. I went to see *den Nasenjosef*, he was very famous, the Joseph-of-Noses, because I had this big nose. Now there was an anti-Semitic paper and in the paper it told about a girl from Osnabrück that she'd had *den Synagogenschlüssel* redone. That was in the paper *der Wächter* and the one who'd had the key to the synagogue trimmed it was me. *Dann haben sie genau gewusst*. It's a small town and people knew exactly where the key was. Me I was disgusted. And mostly embarrassed. And you couldn't complain. After when my daughter had a big nose that she didn't want, she couldn't go and see the *Nasenjosef*, who had been deported, but there was his successor. There was still the *Antisemitismus*. And the big noses we always had them fixed, and the children of the children's noses too even when there is no anti-Semitism.

—Hitler, says my aunt, I thought it's only a year and it's not going to last. But the big nose doesn't just last for a year.

—The Jews, says my mother, were more racist than the racists, but you can't say it, says my mother. With the Poles the German Jews who had a very good position, of course one felt superior.—It is always the poor Poles who came, says my aunt.—No need to spit in our own soup, says my mother.—But I'm not spitting, says my aunt. We always gave them money.—*Ne!Ne!* Not money, says my mother, train tickets. There were always pogroms in Poland. They were a motley bunch, who turned up on our doorsteps, moaning and groaning about how miserable they were. They would come to the consistory. The consistory would give them a train ticket for the next town. Don't repeat it. One mustn't spit on one's own name. Still there was a feeling of caste, or class. Already Frau Engers, although she wasn't Polish, she would talk very loud, she didn't have good manners.—And the Ehrlichs?—Them too. We didn't associate with them.—Horst Engers, says my aunt, he came to see us. I spoke to him, but I didn't invite him. Not just the people of Polish origin nobody associated with them. So in this little German community there were castes. Frau Engers too who didn't have good manners. Those big families who had the big stores, they were Omi's school friends and vice versa. The school friends it was the big families who had the big stores.

—There was another group, that was the lawyers. They didn't mix with the *Kaufleute*, the merchants. Only Omi crossed the line with Frau Engers who made hats however but she had a small business and her husband was only a traveling salesman for pharmaceutical and Dutch products.

This friendship between two people 100 percent different and also the background not being the same, only Omi could do that. Says my mother.

Children were seen and not heard at table in the best families. Except us, Omi's children. Aunt Here blames her that the children we speak at table. But Omi tells her sister: So who do I speak to then? There were even castes at table. But that doesn't go out of this room, says my mother.

AND NOW LOOK WHAT HAS COME TO PASS in this Maternity room, only a few years after the nose crisis, a child with the key to the synagogue sawn off at birth, will wonders never cease. Adam? She murmurs. All the while musing on the semantic ghost of the verb *to come* in its role of ancillarized auxiliary, it's that he hasn't yet come into being, he who is come. She too begins to dissolve a little in the room, a distancing of herself misting her, yesterday was in another time, the join won't take, the relationship between her and Adam of the pug nose who bears the name of George her father growing stronger with every moment, everything is farther away and everything is closer than everything, they are under the influence.

Or is it maybe that it's the cut, the impossible cut with her father that has finally at long last taken place?

'George' she murmurs, 'George' she bursts out, it's the first time she calls the name of her dead father, 'George!' George gives a feeble blink of his feebly slanted eyes, coming back from having come from afar.

What could be less improbable—the Wheel of Time spins on its axis, here comes the Absentee.

I don't know how many children I had. *If* I *had* some how many I have. Kept, lost, put away, eaten up. And how many I may still have, find, lose abandon especially, refuse to have them in my house but not in my heart of hearts. How to add up the living and the dead, the ephemeral and the enduring. Neither addition, nor subtraction, nor succession. I never mention my son the dead to avoid any misunderstanding for if it is more or less true that one of my sons is deceased, he is none the deader for that, it is truer that I never had nor lost my elder son. The truth of the matter is neither recognizable nor thinkable, nor separable from me. He is hardy, he is mixed into my circulation, he is entwined with my roots, forgotten to my memory, furtive, barely sketched, what remains is his wilted smile, his portrait jaundiced at birth, growing yellower and yellower, as the months went by, for he ate nothing but carrots. That too was a surprise, a chagrin, and relief: nothing but carrots and never a drop of any milk. As long as I tried to feed him milk as a child like any other, he brought it all up, all milk was a threat of death. Mother's milk cow's milk powdered milk Nestlé milk, Pelargon milk, poison milk, assassinated with milk. When he had no more skin on his buttocks nor on his back, the flesh peeled off, flayed, him dangling by needles to the drip, my horrible-to-contemplate larva, a baby bunny hunted down by his family which orders the worm to about-face I no longer knew whom to want to die me too pinned to the pinup, and nostalgia for the placental time when without blows and wounds we were one and the same blood.

I have a son and another son. The one who talks and the one to whom I have never said I. Already in the room in Sainte-Foy, he is the-one-who-is-not-there, in person. Of all my children he is the only no-one-in-person. The family hero. The key to my interior synagogue, the director of my faith. All without a word. The simple saint. And my breasts bound till the milk dries up. When I understood that the infant blithely given the name of George, and Adam, and Lev, was my unconscious loss, my loss of consciousness, and that that loss was the key to my life, and that I was twenty-two, I set out. Me and the Absentee, his pale and yellow little impersonage.

—This infant has mongoloid features says the Catholic pediatrician on his way out.

—That? It's a mongolian. Better to put him out of his misery, your little patient, you'll see. A vegetable. At best an animal. I've got one in the building. Can't keep his head up. I attached it to a plank, says the Jewish pediatrician to the midwife my mother.

Eve our mother looks up the mongolian in the dictionary. It's her first. Thus Asia the immemorial comes back.

From Tatar, Ulaanbatar, small bare-backed horses faster than the wind gobble up the fat of the steppes mixed with little children whose cheeks are rubbed red and their gallop has just flickered out panting behind the square window of Sainte-Foy. The Tatar sorcerers and sorceresses croak at the slant-eyed window. From very far they had smelled seen the odor of us and ours. They want to sing:

Chorus of Mongolians
We the mongolians
If a mother lifts us up
In her arms she holds the supernatural continents
On the map you won't find us
She is lifting God's trial-pieces

We the mongolians we look like God and like nobody, neither ugly nor mean we are orphans we belong to no parent

Mongolian to mongolian we repeat ourselves.

These days no one says *mongolian* anymore,

Mongolian, it's not a nice word. *Downs syndrome* is better, less noticeable, less crude, less believed and believing, it's more scientific and less god.

—*Down's syndrome, preferred medical terminology*. Henceforth there are no more mongolians.

We are mummified silkworms in an abandoned cocoonery on the road to Ulaanbaatar. We are larval angels crusting the rungs of the ladder sunk in the bottom of the Dead Sea.

On the paper our letters washed away by the storm
Who will read the message?
When? When ever?
If a mother lifts us to her lips in tears
We cry—an!—an! and at best—man!

In Algeria during the World War, there was also a substitution in 1940 and in correct terminology on the part of sensitive souls, not Jews but from one day to the next it was *Israelites preferable*, instead of Arab *preferred terminology indigenous peoples*, instead of 'I want' better to say 'I should like.'

We the mongolians if somebody stares at us
We make them yearn for the lost country
Stones carved in the homeland in the days of God
Our eroded faces resemble the face of time passing
Promising age with its furrows

We are the vaguely children without schoolbags. At the door to the schoolhouse which everyone enters except for us, we wave our webbed hands

Around the air where the silver ball slips from our grasp, for us the ball goes too fast we wake too late to catch it alive still, we are sick about that.

But if someone dead is buried in the family we do not keep his soul from returning to roost in our gills, for we have no right (or wrong) age. We are nice nice nice!

He's an emperor without dominion, an emperor who draws from his misery of human rabbitry an absolutely enigmatic empire exercised over any person who ever once lifts him up off the ground. Should an unwary person take him in her arms, right away a spell is cast over her. The attachment is worse than a magic potion. Some innocent vampire hides in this rabbit: the absolute authority of the rabbitlamb born for the sacrifice and who asks nobody where the lamb is that will take his place. But it's a lamb that can't stand on its own feet. Bumpety-bump up the Moriah slope, it's a long steep climb. How many years?

One year and fifteen days more or less.

But naturally starting out one doesn't know when and how it's going to end, this trial. Everything having been already decided, all one has to do is keep on, slowly and surely, to the finish, without an idea and without an opinion.

Besides when the infant George was already deceased and buried in the Saint-Eugene Jewish Cemetery, my son remained alive as long as the news of the event hadn't reached me, which took place just before the birth of his brother, my living son. 'Two weeks ago,' says my mother, turning up on the dot for the next one. About a fortnight ago, ten days or fourteen does it matter, one is at the crossroads, dead already alive still a little less dead than dead, but for the record preferred terminology: *deceased*. Right after the news my son the following takes his place in the shredded booklet. But even then. Until this morning I never read those papers. 1 had never read the news. There was no date.

Death does not interest my mother the midwife. The news of the disappearance of persons close to her does not reach her.

—Omi's brothers and sisters who disappeared in the concentration camp, when did you hear?

She has no idea.

—The death of little George?—What can I say?—But you were there?

She never manages to have been there. Years later, the death hasn't happened yet. Maybe never. Death exists? She'd rather not know.

Letter to my son to whom I have never written a letter

My love, to whom I have never declared my love,

I write in the house I had built because of you, in haste for you and against you while Eve our mother was looking after you, I was building I wasn't writing anymore, instead of poems, I was building I responded to your arrival with stones for the time of times, I welcomed you, I fended you off, in haste I raised a house to hold us and to keep us apart, I built the house to which you have never come. A house finished on 1 September 196– on the day you too were done.

I never think of the origins of this house born of your birth. When I knew your name overnight I ceased to write.

I write in this house that I built never to write again.

I inherited this house in which I write to you about your interminable passage.

I'll thou you, I'll conjure you, I'll lure you from your hidden nest.

In this brief truce of an I'll, I'll take in my arms the ghost of the flayed lamb.

As I was writing I felt his cheek grate against my lips.

—Well, that one won't be needing the *Nasenjosef* says my aunt.

—He looks a little strange to me says my mother. I asked a friend of your father, a Jewish pediatrician. At the time I hadn't a clue.

—It's a mongolian, I'm saying it to you, but don't tell the family.

—It's not the sort of thing you say. All mongolians look alike. Another embarrassment. So I said: It's my grandson and the friend never got over his anger at me.

All these distinctions, says my mother, Jews too, they make distinctions.

The word: *distinction*. Omi was very distinguished. Right up to George's birth, she was the most distinguished member of the family. How does one distinguish distinction? And now, the one who's distinguished, it's my son the mongolian. But Omi came from such a good family she was admitted to the lodge of woman Freemasons, even if she was friends with Frau Engers. She was well brought up but it didn't bother her that Frau Engers wasn't well brought up. The German Jews with the Polish Jews, one feels superior, it always bothered me this feeling of caste, I was already for Europe in 1925 with Fraulein von Längeke our German teacher but afterward what bothered me most it's when the Nazis started giving the impression of making the same distinctions but of course that was just a pretense. The consistory was in prison but they thought only Polish Jews were deported as if they were more Jewish for being Polish and they more German albeit Jewish thus both more and less Jewish at once.

And only dogs with three legs are abandoned on the First of May who being cut dogs are less than dogs therefore no longer dogs and more obviously abandonable.

But all this depends on how you look at it and is secondhand.

Translation by Beverly Bic Brahic

The Blue Chair
A Literary Report on Dementia in America

Frederik Tygstrup

Abstract
The blue chair is where the father of the protagonist siblings in Jonathan Franzén's novel *Corrections* ends his life; a comfortable, restful and utterly ugly chair, the only piece of furniture of his own acquisition in an up-marked American suburban home; and the last confine of a mishap existence that has lost its directions through forced retirement and soon escapes into precocious dementia. From having been a marginal and rather inconspicuous disease, dementia, especially in the guise of Alzheimer's disease, has become one of the major challenges to health-care in the industrialised world during the last 20 years or so. This article examines some of the ways in which the rapidly increasing number of patients with the diagnosis of dementia is reflected and negotiated in contemporary American fiction. Through a reading of three novels, Amy Tan's *The Bonesetters Daughter*, Chuck Palahniuk's *Choke* and Franzén's *The Corrections*, all published in 2001, it is discussed how the phenomenon of dementia highlights and expresses some more general features in contemporary culture, especially the changing role of cultural memory in a uniformed culture of consumption, the blurring boundaries between the real and the imaginary in a mediatised society, and the transformation of generational authority in a culture where youthfulness is idealised. On the basis of these readings, it is argued that the role of literature in relation to the disease of dementia can be seen not only as a phenomenological first-person approach to the experience of patients and relatives, but also as a diagnosis of some cultural predicaments supporting the spread of the clinical syndrome, and not least some strategies for coping with the disease in this expanded cultural context.

Key Words: American literature; coping strategies; cultural memory; dementia; generational authority; society

*****

> 'The chair was overstuffed, vaguely gubernatorial. It was made of leather, but it smelled like the inside of a Lexus. Like something modern and medical and impermeable that you could wipe the smell of death off easily, with a damp cloth, before the next person sat down to die in it.'

The chair – thoroughly comfortable and intensely ugly – turns up in Jonathan Franzen's novel *The Corrections*, and is the only piece of furniture in the tidy middle-class family home acquired by the protagonist's father himself. It was quickly relegated to the basement, which remained the elderly father's location of choice after retiring and being himself relegated to the home that had never been his domain. He lives in a shrinking world: while his outer field of operations is reduced from the city streets and working life to the home, the mall and occasional senior outings, to the hobby room and idleness, his mental operations are also reduced by quickly onrushing dementia. Steadily more confused, aggressive and unreasonable in his basic dealings with his surroundings, he is ever more attached to his blue chair – an idiosyncratic fixed point in a dissolving world – until it, too, becomes indifferent and forgotten in the ruinous darkening.

Dementia is one of the fastest-spreading ailments today. According to the United States Department of Health, Education and Welfare, the number of Americans diagnosed with Alzheimer's disease has doubled since 1980 to more than four million, and it is estimated that there will be between 12 and 16 million in 2050. The main treatment efforts are aimed at care and training, and the cost of care is steeply increasing. In the US alone, it is expected that costs will jump from 2000's $30 billion to $50 billion in 2010.

The condition can only be precisely diagnosed once it is too late, that is, by means of a brain dissection, but it does have a relatively recognizable clinical profile. Treatment possibilities are limited, and various medicines have been tried without noteworthy success. Research into the disease's development is intensive but scattered; work is being done on neurobiological explanations, genetic factors and lifestyle factors, but basically the causes are unknown. The most significant risk factor for Alzheimer's is age. Thus, one of the most widespread explanations for the disease's sharp increase is the increased life expectancy in the industrialized world, where better living conditions and medical care mean that more people are living to a relatively advanced age. It is estimated that about half of nursing home residents suffer from Alzheimer's or related conditions.

On this basis, one can almost speak of an Alzheimer's epidemic. Until around 1980 it was not given very high priority in public health policy or pharmaceutical industry investing and occupied only a modest place in ordinary public awareness. Naturally, dementia was a known disease, which just like senility has always been a common diagnosis, but it has only become mapped and seriously visible in the culture in the past 25 years.

If one considers Alzheimer's along with some other contemporary 'big' diseases – cancer, AIDS, diabetis, heart disease – and their cultural meaning, several differences leap to mind. Feared diseases are feared for different reasons. The above-mentioned mythological diseases represent the threat of a short life and painful death as their common characteristics, while being linked to risk factors in the individual's lifestyle: smoking causes cancer; sexual promiscuity causes AIDS; unhealthy eating causes diabetis; lack of exercise causes cardio-pulmonary diseases, etc. In both respects dementia stands apart. It is neither deadly nor, presumably, painful for the body and consciousness enduring it, insofar as the continuous decrease in mental functions is presumably not experienced *from within* as a disease. This does nothing to discourage intensifying fear of the disease as a sort of death-like loss of selfhood while living, a basically sinister dissociation of body and mind. This is a sophisticated fear, not of experiencing the disease, but of having it without experiencing it, just as it is a fear of being a burden for others, of disgracing oneself without knowing it. The psychological and social adaptation to disease that is so significant in the case of the other named diseases – recognition, acceptance, the *dignified* confrontation with the disease – becomes plainly irrelevant to dementia. Furthermore, it is a disease that is evidently undeserved; as no lifestyle-related elements in its development have yet been identified, it comes back to the one: being old enough. It is the prize that awaits the person who avoids or survives cancer, AIDS diabetis, arterial sclerosis – the reversal of success in a final fiasco.

In other words, dementia is a disease that mobilizes cultural metaphors and conceptions completely different from the usual. Loss of self, loss of dignity, having to be a burden for others – and finally institutionalization, being kept many more years as a ghostly spectre, the self's envelope without a self. To imagine oneself as demented is to imagine oneself as another: oneself in flesh and blood, but unable to recognize and take responsibility for that self. An unwieldy self-image: to see oneself not as suffering, but as slavering; and to have spent one's life taking care of the body only to turn it over to another, the demented alter ego. Negotiating the thorny distinction between having and being a body is dramatized here: the body one was lives on in the care of and to the despair of others, while the body one had is beyond one's control.

Another recurrent theme in the discussion of dementia is how the family, social network and health care and nursing home staff conduct their social and professional contacts with a demented person. The central problem is naturally that the suspension of basic recognition and normal, mutual social acknowledgement inevitably skews interpersonal relations. Relatives stop occupying the positions they have filled through years of family history and intimacy. In the demented person's reflection they are reduced to extras in an absurd mental drama whose sense they cannot fathom, and consequently the former ignores the good will and sacrifice they manifest. Concurrently, there is an inevitable reification of the demented person as a living but unpredictable body and a corresponding intensification of feelings of abandonment and desperation on the part of the entourage. For close relatives the result is an extreme and disconcerting experience of being strangers to the elder, and conversely having to see him as an object (which still does not recognize its own status as an object of well-intentioned care), and partly as an image of a loved and close-at-hand person, which it resembles without being, the same way a corpse resembles a person no longer present. This corpse-like similarity is presumably one of the most imposing ways in which the sorrow and desperation of dealing with the demented person gives way to an ominous invocation of death and its proximity to the life that indefatigably beats on in the alien body.

Even as dementia puts these basic questions of identity into play, it affects some of the ways in which we currently conceive the course of a human life. Since the industrial revolution and triumph of the bourgeoisie human life has been thought of in conjunction with use value and productivity, and for just as long old age has been a problem: the old, who no longer contribute to societal reproduction by giving sage counsel, divining the weather and taking care of chickens and children, have become redundant in and to themselves. But in that age when the elderly are no longer worn out from industrial work and poverty and put to impotent rest in nursing homes, and when they are richer than ever, old age has become a new realm of utopic freedom. The 'third age' has become the focal point of the new, broad middle class's dream of freedom and experiences for which there is no room in the still more busy productive years, just as a lucrative market segment has developed for historical travel, cruises, events, elderly housing and all sorts of accessories, not least pension plans and similar financial products. In the late twentieth-century production boom, old age – along with childhood – became a crucial potential market in a heated economy.

The advent of a 'third age' reflects a real new realm of freedom. It is marketed as freedom to harvest a reward that will free us from the type of life that has ruled most of our existence even as it binds us to it as effective consumers. But it also indicates an actual and relatively indefinite potential for existential realization, whereby a long, healthy old age opens the possibility of uninterestedly pursuing – so to speak – individual goals unconnected to any usual use-value calculation and naturally crucial to be turned to account for their consumer potential.

Dementia stands out as an illness that by virtue of these cultural and economic factors has the potential to become a 'big' disease with massive cultural awareness and a correspondingly great franchising potential.

Dementia draws attention as a new threat corresponding to a new biopolitical situation, almost as a type of historical irony that turns the notion of a 'third age' into a grim double image: to have finally achieved the care-free age, free from worry, free to enjoy, to do things for the sake of the doing, only now in a radically different and distorted mode – without possessing the awareness that could set the freedom in perspective against the background of that hard-working and duty-driven life, which would produce the notion of enjoyment. The third age's freedom is both radicalized and negated: it is a radical freedom in its unrestricted regression and a freedom that is no longer capable of being measured against the constraints from which it should be an escape.

The new cultural situation: the new biopolitical potential of old age, and the new threats to it, which allow the inherent contrasts in the new old age scenario to come insistently forward, have naturally not evaded the attention of contemporary literature. Without looking in any systematic way, I have recently come across three new American novels that in different ways deal with the phenomenon of dementia and explore its wealth of realistic and imaginary resources: Amy Tan's *The Bonesetter's Daughter*[1], Chuck Palahniuk's *Choke*[2] and Jonathan Franzen's previously mentioned *The Corrections*[3], all published in 2001. In the following I will examine how specific themes associated with dementia and Alzheimer's disease are developed in these novels, concentrating on figures of *memory*, *community* and *self-determination*, in order to outline some of the traits of the disease's profile in contemporary culture.

A common characteristic of Tan, Palahniuk and Franzen's novels is their point of departure in the relatives' experience and the various forms of discomfort they encompass. The protagonists are all children of dementia sufferers – two mothers and one father – and they all become involved in different ways in the dissolution that is not only personal, but financial as well. An important motif in all of the novels is the enormous economic burden of buying acceptable care for a demented person in the United States, along with a number of cultural and identity-related processes that go along with treating the disease. The novels not only present gripping accounts, in different ways, of the catastrophes the disease brings into the lives of those affected, they also investigate how the disease initiates a cultural self-reflexion, an examination of the resources available to our civilization for dealing with this alien experience, and finally an examination of what kind of image of us appears in the distorting mirror of the disease.

Amy Tan's novel is a framed story, composed of two levels. The first level, which opens and closes the novel, is the story of the Chinese-American Ruth, who is in her forties and leads a normal American life. She works as a ghost writer of popular science lifestyle books and lives with a man and his teenage daughter, and the novel begins as a delicate portrait of daily life with a focus on the many small perceptions, concerns and normal doings that characterize it. Ruth's Chinese mother LuLing occupies an obscure place therein, as a somewhat alien old lady, who despite a long life in the US maintains Chinese habits, postures and ways of speaking, which are not experienced by the daughter as a cultural legacy, but rather more as a personal idiosyncracy. Ruth has been largely raised as an American and thinks of herself as such, with the Chinese as a chance nuance in a culturally mixed society. But the mother's incipient senility eventually brings about a change. Gradually, LuLing becomes more Chinese; apace with losing her grip on reality and beginning to falter over the familiar, no longer knowing how to grasp situations she has managed on countless occasions – mixing up routines, appointments and times and losing the immediate sense of reality – another person begins to show up in her. It is sometimes said that the demented return to childhood, not just because of their lack of ability to handle everyday demands and habits is childlike, but also because early memories, influences and character-shaping experiences emerge, possibly because the loss of short-term memory leaves room for the old elementary ruts of consciousness, or because the weakened censor of consciousness allows the character-shaping primal incidents in remembered life to emerge in a freely associative and chaotic way. In LuLing's case, however, it is not just a childhood universe that begins to find expression – it is a Chinese child's universe. The alienation that characterizes the demented person's behavior and mental universe – the childlike, atemporal, unreasonable and illogical – are in this case doubly alien: not just incomprehensible thoughts, words and actions, but incomprehensible thoughts, words and actions in Chinese.

The immigrant who reverts to childhood is not just picking up the submerged motives of abnormal behavior in another time, but also from an entirely different place. It is a recognized clinical and therapeutic hypothesis that treatment of demented people of a so-called other cultural backgrounds in the future will demand a lot of resources, simply because dementia allows expression of rudiments of cultural baggage that are even more difficult to relate to.

In Amy Tan, Ruth's struggle to reach her every day more demented mother, to hold onto contact and dialogue – which takes up more and more of her resources and leads to the collapse of steadily greater parts of the rest of her life – is also a struggle to enter a past and a story that up until now has been irrelevant and at very best anecdotal. In a certain sense the struggle becomes one to roll back an overly successful cultural integration, and thus a struggle to reclaim cultural memory. This effort points into the frame narrative's second level, a story within the story, which takes up about half of the novel. LuLing has at an earlier moment entrusted a large Chinese manuscript to Ruth, recounting her dramatic youth and the family history in

China before and after the revoltion and during the Second World War. Ruth has not given the notebook any special attention, having at times read just single sentences and sat down to read it in order to learn Chinese without having got farther than the intention. But afterwards, as her mother becomes lost in odd family historical intrigues and obscure allusions, the manuscript becomes important to her and she finally arranges for a translation. As mentioned, the framed text occupies a large portion of the novel, and is in itself a fascinating narrative fusing existential, historical and mythological elements into a portrait of a Chinese time and life endowed with an alien, sometimes poetic and sometimes brutal universe with an internal cohesion that is not just fascinating in itself, but also points out some traits of the demented LuLing's worldview, which would otherwise have to be chalked up to her dementia.

The novel's two parts thus merge in an understanding process whereby Ruth's attempt to reach her mother in her increasing darkness can now draw upon an intimacy she had not been able to deliver in their American life together. On the other hand, this does not involve any facile therapeutic notion of fighting the disease through understanding and cultural insight; the disease is irreversible and loss of contact is the unavoidable perspective. It is more a tribute to writing – constantly underscored in a respect for calligraphy and the writer's self-imposed (or tradition-imposed) discipline in order to meet oneself in the writing. In this sense there is more insistence on the harmony between LuLing's manuscript and Ruth's than on the written accounts' instrumental application in the therapeutic situation. They are two women trying to find themselves and the small girls they were, in the writing. And thus in the final instance it is a defence of literary culture – the Chinese and the (declining) Western – as the locus where identities can be conceived and meet.

In Amy Tan's work, the cultural context in which dementia is about to become one of the central folk illnesses is implicitly outlined: a culture in which individual cultural memory – the sensory and reflective experience of being a little girl in a particular place – is increasingly discounted, and heterogeneous life forms are grouped and homogenized in effective and generic customs, creating effective and inviolable social conventions, in which idiosyncratic and locally conditioned modes of constituting and understanding the self slip out of circulation. It would be cynical to call the disease a remedy for cultural forgetting of the individual character development's specificity. Nonetheless, the disease appears, despite its fatality, as a manifestation of that forgetting and the encounter with it as a salutary awareness of the resource that literary culture has been and can still be: the disciplined awareness of what constitutes identity formation, which is too easily overlooked amidst the models of subjectivity produced in a present-oriented culture.

Amy Tan's novel opens a poetic universe of individual meaning through an alert sensing and reflection in the confrontation with the disease. Therein are both an existential strategy for dealing with that forgetting that grows into one's life with the disease and a cultural strategy for opposing the cultural forgetting of which the alarming growth in dementia has its distorted reflection. Chuck Palahniuk's *Choke* operates in the same field, where declining cultural memory and the nearly epidemic spread of dementia go hand in hand, but his angle of attack is diametrically opposite. Here it is not a question of remonstrating against the disease, but of deploying a snearing radicalization – gruesome, baroque, funny and scary. The premise is structured similarly to Tan's: a demented mother brought to a nursing home, and a son, Victor, who attempts to maintain sort of a contact with her and who must pay for the costly care. Their family history is chaotic; Victor spent most of his childhood in various foster families while his mother lived like a caricature of a 1960s outlaw, alternately in jail, on the lam, and generally in a hurry. Her worldview combines anarchism and paranoia, a longing for freedom and mistrust of 'the system', and her crimes consist mainly of various forms of sabotage against the American middle class's new frantic consumerism. When she is on the loose she gladly abducts the boy from his changing foster families and drifts around for a while teaching him the pitfalls for human freedom that constitute organized society. In other words, Victor is not close to his mother, but has in his nature a fundamental acceptance of her limitless social criticism, not as an articulated critical awareness, but rather a combination of quasi-intuitive insight into the modern US as a huge, grotesque consumption-stimulated bluff and an odd anarchic will to realize the world of egoism and consumption – no longer according to the American dream as an attractive object of desire, but more as a kind of devil-may-care letting oneself be swept along. The critical verve no longer contains the notion of a better life, but a cynical indulgence in the kicks that this life offers.

Victor does not live the American life, he acts out on a whim the various roles that life invites him to as a seedy actor on a stage he neither takes seriously nor rejects. His profession underscores this logic: he works at a kind of historical theme park, an artificial 18th century village whose employees are dressed and trained to create the illusion of colonial America of 1734 for the edification of uninterested school children and photo-snapping tourists, while they themselves are mainly occupied with smoking pot, conducting erotic intrigues and keeping a straight face while pulling the legs of their distracted audience with improbable tales. It is a bizarre but good and genuine job that yet has nothing to do with reality, but is a sort of illusion number on a precarious margin between entertainment and education, while being an impotent simulation of historical memory – what is left of history in contemporary consumer culture. He does not work in a society that has a history, but rather in a society of spectacle, as Guy Debord called it. Only his job is not sufficient to defray the costs of his mother's nursing home, so he has found a supplementary source of income, faking choking fits while dining in restaurants. There is always someone, he has found, who will intervene – a man or woman of action who will turn him round, bend him over, and save him by getting him to spit up that stuck bit of food. And the hero is moved, feeling suddenly meaningful. The savior will adopt him, think about him, follow along with his life, exchange Christmas cards and not least send a check when he has problems. Victor has systematized his restaurant visits and correspondence and thus can pay the $3000 per month for his mother's stay at St. Anthony's Care Center. The grotesque trick, from which the novel takes its name, is another offshoot of the society of spectacle's imaginary economy, an act that provides the hero du jour with an unadulturated sense of reality, an opportunity to intervene and save a human life right in the middle of the desert of bad images. This, then, is the source of the perverse debt: not the being saved, but being given the chance to save. It is a momentary awakening from televised reality, 'You know, real people pretending to be fake people with made-up problems being watched by real people to forget their real problems'.[4]

These inside-out short circuits between a staged fantasy and a real economy, which consistently call into question our ideas about living in a reality and being able to fantasize on its solid foundation, also encompass the book's third large theme, sex. Victor is a clinically diagnosed sexaholic, even enrolled in a treatment group, though it primarily serves as an exchange of tips and experiences, and the book is constantly sprinkled with elements of an obstinately realized pornographic worldview – every bit as tiresome as the majority of pornographic fictions from Sade to Houellebecq, but not infrequently disarmingly funny in its ongoing explication of pornographic scenarios' pale rationality. Whereas the theme park and choking act consistently play out the imaginary virtualizing of the real, the disenchanting sexuality completes the mixture by making the closed world of fantasy real, not as a utopian project, but as a tired clinical syndrome.

On the basis of this view of reality, it becomes self-evidently difficult to pass an unambiguous judgement on the Alzheimer's-smitten patients' weakening sense of reality. Their world of forgetting, bodily regression and hallucinated fantasy is not necessarily much different from the American reality as lived by Victor and his contemporaries. At first Palahniuk describes the nursing home in the same wondering, cauistical mode he uses for the surrounding society.

> Here at St. Anthony's, they show the movie *The Pajama Game* every Friday night, and every Friday all the same patients crowd in to see it for the first time.
>
> They have bingo, crafts, visiting pets.
>
> They have fireproof bibs that cover you from your neck to ankles so that you don't set fire to yourself while you smoke. They have Norman Rockwell posters. A hair dresser comes twice a week to do your hair. That costs extra. Incontinence costs extra. Dry cleaning costs extra. Monitoring urine output costs extra. Stomach tubes.
>
> They have lessons every day in how to tie your shoe, how to button a button, snap a snap. Buckle a buckle. Someone will demonstrate Velcro. Someone will tell you how to zip your zipper. Every morning, they tell you your name. Friends who've known each other sixty years get reintroduced. Every morning.
>
> These are doctors, lawyers, captains of industry, who, day to day, can't master a zipper anymore. This is less teaching than it is damage control. You might as well try to paint a house that's on fire.[5]

The unreality and meaninglessness here appears only slightly magnified, but not significantly different from the rest of Victor's life.

In his eccentric existence, which reacts to the growing fuzziness in the distinction between reality and images, life and fantasy, with a radicalizing combination of social life as an act and acting as a way of life, Victor soon finds a way to deal with the nursing home's disquieting world of appearances. It is in the nature of the case that none of the elders can recognize or identify him, least of all his mother, but they are all enormously interested when a rare visitor comes into the home, and come rolling and shuffling out of the corners, each one taking him for a character out of their very own fading fantasy universe. And naturally he may play along; it is of no use to explain himself, so he rather attempts as best he can to live up to the roles' expectations. 'Here I get to be all things to all women'.[6] He starts keeping books on each individual role, not least the complicated one as one of his mother's case workers, where she zealously keeps an eye out for the details: the number of children, makes of cars, the summer house, most important cases…All of the elders have their own scripts that he memorizes and improvises from. For that reason he becomes a beloved person in the place, or rather appreciated, not beloved; an ongoing occurrence is that the senile residents choose to let him take on the role of some hated person who has in different ways offended, cheated, insulted or affronted them. The dream of having a genuine social relationship in the midst of the nursing home's disinfected termination ambiance unavoidably converges in an outbreak of aggression. Being wronged becomes the final human feeling.

This gloomy atmosphere pervades the entirety of Palahniuk's picture of 21st century old age. Nonetheless, the book's emotional tune is not in fact gloomy; it is more baroque, and basically funny with its constant, well-turned one-liners, which unsentimentally chronicle wretchedness. In this meaningless high mood the book – and its protagonist-narrator – seems to have found its own indomitable survival strategy, as if it had long ago abandoned the ambition of elucidating and evaluating the contemporary conditions of life. Rather, it bets on exaggeration and simulation, which constantly go too far to catch up with and outdo the absurdity evidenced by daily life and eventually become a way of life encouraging realization of a certain short-lived feeling of freedom. Every now and then, exaggeration and travesty go so far that they can almost reach something that can no longer be integrated into the common halluncinatory sense of reality. It is perhaps a touch of that freedom Victor's mother dreamed of in her day, though not as a whole other world, but rather as the blossoming of a mad seed in the great fantasy factory of contemporary American culture. In that sense there is a suggestion of a rapprochment of Victor and his demented mother in the nearly Jesuit strategy of vanquishing the burdensome contemporary culture with its own methods. It is not a regular, existentially comforting rapprochement, which dementia excludes in all circumstances, but a meeting on the edge, a shared or at least parallel transgression, whereby the demented one becomes a final instructor of how to accommodate oneself with a measure of autonomy to the raving collective madness.

The cultural diagnosis of the fate of community in an age of an intensified and present-fixated world of images- is, in Palahniuk's hands, cheery without being uplifting. Jonathan Franzen's *The Corrections* has something of the same touch and mood about it, though the tone is completely different. Whereas *Choke* has the raw verve of a cartoon or cult film, *The Corrections* is written more in the tradition of the modern family novel from Thomas Mann to Don DeLillo. The story of the demented father is but one element in the novel's broad sketch of a family history through the last generation, with a focus on its three children and their growth to the present, where they are middle-agers burrying their father. Nonetheless, the father and the parents' home is the hub of the tale, uniting the three children's stories. By virtue of that, the part of the novel dealing with dementia is less focused on the manifest disease than on its gradual development. The description of the father and his illness stems from the presumably crucial terminal day of his working life as a railroad engineer and the beginning of his retired life, which he is totally unprepared to take charge of. Of his former life we see only sketches from an external perspective, the children's view of the parents and their more or less comprehensible – if spontaneously recognized – behavior.

The family's life has been significantly conducted on premises that were structurally the father's, centered on his not particularly interesting or lucrative but proper and respectable work. He has, like most middle-class parents of his generation, possessed a seldom exercised yet nonetheless indisputable authority. The children's love for him is not significantly tied to any personal capacities or character traits, but rather to the security and consistency of his presence. By his side is the mother, who after a long life in the shadows thanks to convention and necessity is looking forward to retired life, which is also a turning point in the power structure: now the man is back in the home, her domain, incapable of managing his time or keeping up his life rhythms, left to her daily routines, which are formed after the most common clichés of happy seniors, homey leisure activities, children and grandchildren (preferably successful and bright), suburban sociability and travel – above all the cruise, the ultimate good as envisioned by the American middle class. It is under this new regime that he retires to the basement, the lonely workroom and the blue chair. And there he withdraws, at first into various infirmities, and finally into full-blown dementia. In the perspective of the novel's premise, dementia is not a disease that strikes one, but rather a condition that sets in where a place has been prepared for it, a vacuum that awareness and ingenuity cannot bring into life, where awareness must thus shrink, so to speak, to adjust itself to the vacuity.

In the chidren's perspective his life has been an exercise in pointlessness, lack of imagination, faith in authority and habit. But there is, nonetheless, a personality that they inevitably love encapsuled in that grey life. Yet their love remains particularly objectless when the structures holding that personality together disintegrate in the minor catastrophe of retirement and the permanent catastrophe of dementia. There is suddenly so infinitely little to hold onto: an emotional quality only held up by conventional structures that lie partly in ruin. At the end of the sequence it becomes clear to the daughter:

> [S]he had never really known her father. Probably nobody had. With his shyness and his formality and his tyrannical rages he protected his interior so ferociously that if you loved him, as she did, you learned that you could do him no greater kindness than to respect his privacy.[7]

Thus a melancholic, contradiction-ridden situation is sketched out. On the one hand is a father who in his simultaneously humble and authoritarian character type can only handle love at a certain distance, who has elevated reassuring ritual to a way of life, and on the other a father who by virtue of the same general traits is en route to darkness and dependency, which is to say into pain, exclusively, since they must of necessity lead to a transgression of the limits implied by the first-named characteristics. The contradictoriness is evident and the melancholic tone unavoidably strikes those caught in the play of contradiction. The father can only be loved at a distance, where his autonomy and self-determination are upheld by an old disciplinary order that constitutes his personality, which consequently prohibits his children from showing their love there where it is most needed.

In Franzen dementia is historicized, not in the outer history – the one examined by Tan and Palahniuk in their mapping of the loss of social memory and the generalized collective hallucination – but rather in a history of generations. In the novel, the parents' generation is the one that can achieve the long, prosperous and healthy life, and yet it has based its welfare and health on a disciplined way of life that cannot cope with a long and healthy old age. It lacks the flexibility of consciousness that could confront the third age's freedom, and it cannot deal with the care that accords love an increasing surrender of control of consciousness and bodily functions. In *The Corrections* dementia is portrayed as a process, a gradual surrender, which cannot be accepted, however, by those who have had the possibility of experiencing it over the course of a long and healthy life.

The three novels all consider dementia in the historical context of the contemporary United States, where over the past twenty years dementia has attained the status of a folk-illness on the top-five list of those most feared and costly, in terms of research and health care expenditures. The United States is a forerunner in this respect and also possibly in producing the patterns of cultural understanding and agency that make the syndrome of dementia reverberate in ordinary cultural life, in memory structures, community structures and personality types. Reading Tan, Palahniuk and Franzen, one gets the impression that everything that is feared in the disease is already present on the cultural horizon – that it is an illness that belongs to this culture, as its reverse side, as its truth, its unavoidable companion. And where fighting the disease is not just a question of neurological, dietary and genetic research, but presumably also a question of cultural self-reflection, and thus, of literature.

Translation by Thomas Petruso

Notes

[1] A Tan, *The Bonesetters Daughter*, Flamingo, London, 2001.

[2] C Palahniuk, *Choke*, Doubleday, New York, 2001.

[3] J Franzen, *The Corrections*, Farrar, Straus and Giroux, New York, 2001.

[4] Palahniuk, p. 40.

[5] ibid., pp. 57–58.

[6] ibid., p. 59.

[7] Franzen, p. 526.

Bibliography

Franzen, J., *The Corrections*, Farrar, Straus and Giroux, New York, 2001
Palahniuk, C., *Choke*. Doubleday, New York, 2001.
Tan, A., *The Bonesetters Daughter*. Flamingo, London, 2001.

Henri Michaux in Search of his *Tempo*, or Great Health

Gérard Danou

Abstract
Henri Michaux clearly stated that he painted and wrote 'for his good health'. Yet, due to his weak heart, he suffered from ill-health all his life. However, not heeding medical advice, he did not spare himself for over 80 years. As he put it, his only drug was 'feeling tired'! By means of 'pen strokes', Michaux lay on paper the innumerable aspects of his psycho-somatic suffering, thereby both exorcizing and alchemizing it through the poetic act. His work focusses on the narcissistic self and phenomenological body awareness: 'Cœnesthésie, mare nostrum', he said. But this did not prevent him from having an accurate perception of other people and of the world, at a distance. By an alchemical process, he appropriated and operated a value-transmutation of the scientific and medical languages of the 20th century for his personal use. He, thus, offers an unclassifiable and open-ended poetry, resisting all power abuse of a single interpretation, especially that of the medical world. According to his poetry function, the 'non-breathable becomes breathable and the unlivable becomes livable'. His whole output is an exercise in perfection, medicine for oneself, a Nietzschean healing pedagogy, that is to say 'good health'.

Key Words: Health; literature; Nietzsche; Michaux

*****

> I wanted to draw the consciousness of existing and the flow of time.
>
> Je voulais dessiner la conscience d'exister et l'écoulement du temps.
>
> H. Michaux, *Passages*.

With Henri Michaux (1899-1984), the nineteenth century anatomo-clinical model of the body, based on the study of life starting from the corpse, gives rise to a completely different way of looking at the body, which one can call phenomenological, well before its common obviousness of today. This new approach gained credence with the poet through the appropriation and distortion of all the scientific and medical knowledge of the twentieth century. It has to do with creating a new language, hence to create a rupture, just like Baudelaire wanted to do in 1850 with his book, *Small Prose poems, Petits Poèmes en prose.*

Influenced by Lautréamont (he says, *He believes he is Maldoror,* around 1925), Michaux establishes another major rupture by using poetic and pictorial writings where the word is grasped in its immanent materiality, which does not exclude a certain lyricism or emotion from the matter. However, Michaux wanted to go further, to the point of suppressing the words (he says, *Down with words, À bas les mots*) in order to paint life's film in himself, its flow, its rhythm and its phrasing. The poetic intention, then, is the grasping of his bodily life, its noises, its movements, even its molecular components, which he renames and transfigures to count them at the level of his *Properties, Propriétés,* in a *Space within, Espace du dedans,* that is in painful tension with the outside, with the world and its objects in space that should be tamed but always resist.

His often comic or enigmatic linguistic inventions are, in effect, movements *to disengage himself* (*se dégager*, a verb he is fond of) from the fixed forms. His project is simple: 'painting, composing, writing, that is the adventure of being alive', '*peindre, composer, écrire, voilà l'aventure d'être en vie.*' Writing to 'explore himself', to survey his domains, his properties, the extent and the structure of his macroscopic and microscopic body. Why? Surely 'to make some something of it', '*en faire quelque chose*', because of 'hygiene', '[*par*] *hygiene*', he adds, for his 'health', '*pour sa santé.*' Let us stress this point, it is not poor health [*la petite santé*] that interests him; he does not neglect it, especially since his health was never good due to the cardiac and psychological fatigue he suffered since childhood, but it always remained something *external* to him. Nevertheless, he does not spare himself. His real voyages bear witness to this, in particular, the hundreds of kilometers crossing the Amazon in a canoe under very testing conditions. In 1945 he writes in the Fontaine journal, '*And it is always the thin arm, like a lash, that fights against the mass of the river', 'Et c'est toujours le bras mince comme un cil qui lutte contre la masse du fleuve.*'

Through the relentless work of a fencer, of a fighter against words like Kafka, what he desires is to attain *good health,* [*la grande santé*]. This Nitzschean *good* or *great* health effects a transmutation of value, a turning of disease into its opposite, extending itself into the force of life. As Edelman argues[1], it is to find, 'the appropriate point of view on life and man's place in life', '*le point de vue juste sur la vie et la place de l'homme dans la vie*', in his materiality and his *animality*, because there is only the body. Thus, in *Ecce Homo*[2], Nietzsche argues that great health is being perfectly *conscious of one's destiny, and loving it.* Thus, it is the power of life's affirmation at the present time and up until death. It is a matter of a pedagogy of the *cure* that we also find in Freud (in which one recognizes a certain similarity of outlook [*de regard*] with Nietzsche), and which he puts forward in his 'Considerations on war and on death', '*Considérations sur la guerre et sur la mort*', (1915) and in the beautiful short text, 'Ephemeral destiny', '*Ephémère destinée*' of the same year. We even find it in G. Canguilhem's (1988), 'Pedagogy of the cure', '*Pédagogie de la guérison.*'

1. The Properties of the Body or Praise of the Elementary

The poet's portable laboratory is the materiality of his body perceived as extension, without a break between the psyche and the soma. Consequently, one would prefer formulations like that of Ajuriaguerra (dweller and dwelling place, *habitant et habitacle*), or perhaps Paul Valéry's triad, 'body, mind, world', '*corps, esprit, monde*', or even, 'subject, world, language', '*sujet, monde, langage*'. This body is seen in its atomic, corpuscular bio-molecular aspect, in motion, but also as organized, above all as a neurological apparatus. Michaux always showed considerable interest for neurology (gnosis of the body) and for the psychiatry of his times, of which he read the works.

Since the nineteenth century, as one knows, writers begin to use all means to come closer to madness, which fascinates them. The use of drugs goes largely in this direction, from Quincey and Baudelaire to Michaux. Nevertheless, there is a specificity in the use of drugs in Michaux (an incidental clause in his work). He experimented when nearing the age of fifty and under the medical supervision of his psychiatrist and anthropologist friends. The drugs helped him explore his body's sensorial capacities, to discover in them new aspects that, up to that point, had been neglected or unsuspected: From paying close attention to the faintest tickling sensations, this 'marvelous normal', '*merveilleux normal*', to the 'images of a visionary world', '*images d'un monde visionnaire*' – title of a film he directed (with little success for his taste), where he tried to put his mescaline induced hallucinations into images.

This keen listening to the body, characteristic of somatic practices, this 'cult of the living machine', '*culte de la machine à vivre*', as Valéry calls it, will be, as I mentioned earlier, either sought by an extreme attention to oneself or indirectly revealed by the use of foreign substances. But it may also happen that a small disease (a dental pain, a furuncle, a tendinous rupture, a venereal affection) and especially a fracture[3] (Broken arm, *Bras cassé*) produces an event that is as gripping as it is something to grasp (*autant saissisant qu'à saisir*), not to let pass passively. This accident, the fracture, will then be (as he says, not 'to waste his time doing nothing', '*perdre son temps à ne rien faire*') an object of observation and of translation in poetic and pictorial writing, generally from a distance, even if he sometimes takes notes in the midst of impotence and pain. The experience of the broken right arm, the suffering, the modifications of his bodily structure (he says that he writes and explores his *left-handed being* [*être gauche*]) will give rise to the writing of a text that will be taken up several times with the passing of years, and which represents for Michaux a monumental event from which he will write one poem – a genuine phenomenological experiment [*essai*] of the most stimulating kind.

What are these images? They are drawn from the feelings and perceptions produced by any modification of the body's structure, and whose observation is made possible by relaxation or autohypnosis, by fixing our attention on one segment of the body at rest: heaviness, heat, cold, breathing, the beating of the heart. As Michaux tells us, everyone carries in himself this poïesis *in potentia*. He invites everyone to find his own poetry. This is a lesson of great health indeed. However, not everyone is Michaux...

2. Identity Loss and Metamorphosis

To whom does this cœnesthetic elementary molecular body (*cœnaesthésie mare nostrum,* he says in *Broken arm, Bras cassé*) belong? The subject of enunciation advances under a mask and seldom in the first person. As R. Bellour suggests, the *I* is in the becoming of the *I*. It generally escapes from the subject of enunciation. Thus, there is subjectivity, but rarely is there ever a subject in Michaux. What interests him, as R. Dadoun writes, is being and its *tenuousness*, being at the verge of its effacement, of its extenuation. That is why his characters are thread-like, supple, elastic, light. The blundering character and poet, *Plume*, is Michaux's double, like Chaplin.

Michaux, who passed away in 1984, would have certainly criticized and distorted the last cry of today's neurosciences, *cerebral plasticity*, to his own profit and thus to ours. The term 'plasticity' implies two simultaneous or consecutive movements: to take form and create, or give form. Thus, there is a neuronal inventiveness, which results in an increase in the dendritic activity, that is to say, increase of the synapses connecting the neurological cells. Just as Catherine Malabou does as a philosopher, Michaux would have scoffed, in his own way, not so much at this important concept of neurobiology and its metaphors, but at what is made of it in relation to its presumed synonym, *flexibility*, in the daily discourse of work and of large liberal enterprises. However, plasticity's semantic definition contradicts all rigidity. Flexibility, as a false cognate of plasticity, cuts down its inventive suppleness to retain that first meaning, the imposing of form, the solidification of the fold to the point of exhaustion and rupture. *Managerial board*, this breakable reed!

After reading attentively and completely the best American neurobiologists' essays, and asking herself with some irony, *What to make of our brain? Que faire de notre cerveau?*, Catherine Malabou[4] shows with her great philosophical talent that this approach can only yield 'medical' responses that do not help us at all to *exist*. It is necessary to quote the whole paragraph:

> How can we not see that the only perspective of real progress opened by the neurosciences is that of an improvement of the 'quality of life' by a more effective treatment of the diseases? However we do not want these half-measures of what Nietzsche would rightly call the despairing and feeble logic of a sick man. What we miss *is life, that is, resistance. Resistance is what we want.* Resistance to flexibility, to this ideological standard conveyed, consciously or not, by the reductionist discourse that models and naturalizes the neuronal process in order to legitimate a certain social and political operation.
>
> *Comment ne pas voir que la seule perspective de progrès réel ouverte par les neurosciences est celle d'une amélioration de la 'qualité de vie' par un traitement plus efficace des maladies ? Or nous ne voulons pas de ces demi-mesures, de ce que Nietzsche appellerait justement une logique de malade, désespérante et souffreteuse. Ce qui nous manque*, c'est la vie, c'est-à-dire la résistance. La résistance est ce que nous voulons. *Résistance à la flexibilité, à cette norme idéologique véhiculée consciemment ou non par le discours réductionniste qui modélise et naturalise le processus neuronal afin de légitimer un certain fonctionnement social et politique.*

It could not be said any better. If poetry succeeds in inventing a new language, if it renews the air that we breathe, Michaux argues, it always does it while rebelling against a certain common use of knowledge and discourses. It is a power of *resistance* that also gives him a value of testimony.

A great part of Henri Michaux's work already pioneers the problematic question of the passage from the neuronal to the psychic without scorning, quite to the contrary, neither one nor the other. Thus, the role of poetry is to resist through invention, not through reaction. Poetry is a vital need.

The metaphors of identity, in Michaux, are omnipresent, in motion, in a state of becoming between the three kingdoms, animal, vegetable, and mineral. His pictorial quests for the forms of passage seem to surge from chance, from control in freedom, an Oriental-style letting go [*lâcher-prise oriental*]. However, this lack of formality – which does not mean without form, without contours, but without a known structure – is prepared by a long work of information, curiosity for the most diverse life sciences. He passionately browses dictionaries, encyclopedias, works of science and medicine. He borrows from Hoeckel, this Neo-Darwinist for whom ontogenesis recapitulates phylogenesis. After his voyages in South America and Asia, he reads the ethnologists of his time like Lévy-Bruhl, and the great sociologists, Durkheim and Mauss. Not only does he read them, but as R. Bellour's beautiful work of intertextuality written for the three-tome edition of the Pléiade shows, he copies entire paragraphs from them, and changes them to his own benefit. He makes something else out of them. What he also retains from his ethnological readings (Lévy-Bruhl's *On Primitive mentality, La mentalité primitive*, for example), like from his real voyages, is his use of magic or magic thought [*pensée magique*] (appearance-disappearance), and of a certain animism that opens up toward other logics of thought different from Western rational logic. It is possible in Michaux, as is the case of the animists, to be two different entities at the same time without contradiction: a man and a tortoise for example, a rock and a cloud...

The figures that emerge from his drawings, even if formless, are always faces (he says, *Men, look at yourselves in the paper*). They appear in a perceptual relation that clashes in this faciality against a radical and enigmatic otherness. Sometimes they are obvious metamorphosic figures with anthropomorphic or zoomorphic traces (*Maldoror* is not far), sometimes disturbing and yet familiar (*unheimlich*), giving form to the interior sufferings that are rejected towards the outside (an outside as distressing as the inside) in order to exorcise them. Although this last aspect can be found in Michaux's paintings, it is not the most frequent aspect, nor is it specific to him. Michaux does not make *Art Brut*, like a madman. Perhaps, as his last writings testify, what he seeks above all is the spontaneity of children's drawings. This is why in *Tent Posts, Poteaux d'angle,* he advises us to *unlearn, désapprendre,* that is, to learn differently.

3. The Bestiary of Michaux

In the bestiary of Michaux, without mentioning the marvelous animals he invented (Parpue or Dardelette!) most of all one finds ants. The *cuttle-fish* is also appreciated for its black ink and its capacity for dissimulation. However, the frog holds a special place in Michaux. This is surely due to his reading of Jean Rostand, and Brisset, that literary lunatic who assembled a theory according to which man is a descendant of the frog. Nevertheless, to metamorphose oneself unceasingly is very tiring:

> There are so many animals, so many plants, so many minerals. And I have already been everything so many

> times. But these experiments don't help me. Becoming ammonium hydrochlorate again for the thirty-second time, I still have a tendency to behave like arsenic, and, changed once more into a dog, my night-bird habits always come through.[5]
>
> *Il y a tant d'animaux tant de plantes, tant de minéraux. Et j'ai été déjà de tout et tant de fois. Mais les expériences ne me servent pas. Pour la trente-deuxième fois redevenant chlorhydrate d'ammonium, j'ai encore tendance à me comporter comme de l'arsenic, et redevenu chien, mes façons d'oiseau de nuit perçent toujours. (Mes propriétés,* Vol. I, p. 479*).*

The effacement of identities, or the multiple identities open the borders, refute the binary cleavages, implying a becoming other. Today, people who go through a heart transplant can be compared to certain of Michaux's representations and chimerical montages. Jean-Luc Nancy[6] tells us in his book on heart transplantation that, as an experience of what is foreign, the *niche of being*, [la *niche de l'être*] can dwell in a monstrous character (Canguilhem, says, *marvelous against the grain, but marvelous nonetheless, merveilleux à rebours, mais du merveilleux quand même*) as well as in a thread-like silhouette – the thread of life personified by the thread of writing, which is also an image, thus a pseudo-presence.

4. Scientific Imaginary and the Poetic Imaginary: The Frog Heart or Sum of all the First Beats since the Dawn of Times

Michaux evokes beautiful images of the frog heart and its infinite beats isolated in a liquid. He saw these experiments at school, and in his first year of medicine. Surely, the representations of his cardiac disease, which does not play a role in his fatigue, also play a considerable part in his fascination for the automatism of the heart. Thus in *Tent posts, Poteaux d'angle,*[7] he writes:

> A frog's heart – you have to have seen it, separated from the body, in a test tube where they put it with an appropriate fluid – continuing to beat for days on end and then some. More impressive than in the original chest from where it was extracted – you have to have seen it cut off from everything, but still vigorous, blindly and vainly about its business, dogged, doing its job without hitch or hesitation, beating, beating, beating from now on for no

> one, a real tide-maker, as when in nature on the inside a lowly batrachian it got hooked up to the arteries and veins of an organism, pushing a wave of blood about once per second, corpuscles and globules and the like. From the time of the embryo, the egg, it was on its way, it set things going – author of circulation.
>
> *-Un cœur de grenouille, il faut l'avoir vu, détaché du corps, en un tube de verre où on l'a mis avec un liquide convenable, continuant à battre, des jours durant et davantage. Plus impressionnant que dans la poitrine originelle d'où il fut extrait, il faut l'avoir vu, coupé de tout, mais toujours vaillant, aveuglément et vainement à son affaire, non distrait, accomplissant sans un raté, sans une hésitation son œuvre de battant, battant, battant dorénavant pour personne, faiseur d'une marée régulière comme lorsque dans la nature à l'intérieur d'un modeste batracien il se trouvait abouché aux artères et veines d'un organisme, poussant environ à chaque seconde un flot de sang, d'hématies et de globules... et le reste. Dès l'embryon, dès l'œuf il était en route, il mettait en route, auteur de la circulation.*

Although fascinated by objective knowledge, Michaux transmutes it with his personal view, that of a subjective world whose horizon varies between what is and is not perceived, between the development of a structure and the opening of a zone of indetermination:

> There had to be stubborn ones like it to have succeeded in at making frogs leap everywhere in so many pools and ponds whether they wanted to or not, the slowpokes like the rest *hurled,* carried off by the tireless coach, condemned to go forth – like it or not – to the future: life's secret.
>
> *Il fallait des butés comme lui pour avoir réussi dans tant de mares et d'étangs à faire sauter partout des grenouilles, qu'elles en eussent envie ou non, les traînardes comme les autres, propulsées, emportées par l'entraîneur infatigable, condamnées à aller de l'avant, bon gré mal gré condamnées à de l'avenir, secret de la vie.*

Thus, in observing the heart, two approaches are possible. The first one measures, that is the glance of science which Michaux distorts to the benefit of a perceptual glance, that of an imaginative conscience, filled with wonder, that attaches itself to the form of things like the glance of a child to this isolated heart plunged in a liquid and beating, beating 'all alone.'

5. Michaux and Space-time: Man is Emotionally Faster

Baudelaire felt in his flesh the 'past of the present', which he calls modernity. The main source of his melancholia is the difference between this high-speed social time and his slower personal tempo, which Michaux himself calls physical, psychological, and phenomenological 'fatigue'. After Baudelaire everything goes even faster, and as Michaux points out, man is cut short, *l'homme s'abrège*. Moreover, the new physics, relativity and quantum physics (the 'soluble fish', '*poisson soluble',* of surrealist and Michaux's invisible 'needle fish', '*poisson aiguille*') make it impossible to think of matter and sign as was done before.

In yet another effort by Michaux to attain great health, he writes, *in a time of restlessness, guard your andante.*[8] If the speed of travel increases, Michaux thinks that the body's perceptual impressions would also increase. Honneger confirmed this in music, in the arts, and poetry, Blaise Cendrars, and it was also confirmed in the cinema. In 1925, in one of his first textes, *Chronicle of the pointsman/Chronique de l'aiguilleur,*[9] he uses the mathematical formula of speed. However, instead of writing that it is equal to the ratio of the distance over time, he introduces a qualitative, subjective, and relative aspect to the formula. It is about the poet, about his emotionally affected body measuring itself to space and time by the study of its emotions. Instead of placing the distance as the numerator, he prefers space (E). The ratio becomes the following, Speed is the space traversed, over the time put to traverse it. One is really in Michaux, in his body, in his properties, his poetic and pictorial writing, because as one recalls, he says to us that he 'writes in order to traverse himself',

> The arts reveal the emotive practices of the times: literature and modern music reveal the multiplication, the abbreviation of emotions and representations.
>
> *Les arts révèlent les habitudes émotives d'une époque : la littérature et la musique moderne révèlent la multiplication, l'abrévation des émotions et des représentations*. (Vol. I., p. 14-15)

Emotive speed, he argues, becomes the ratio of emotional space or field of emotions over time employed to traverse it. The employed, *employé* (somewhere between the verb and the noun), is an employee for time, like Charlot's *Modern times, Les Temps modernes*, or Fritz Lang's *Metropolis*. Thus, Michaux transforms quantitative equations into relative, tangible measurements. In the same way, the electrocardiograms that he undergoes with interest in Ecuador give no essential account for his being heart [*être cœur*]. The poet's body does not cease to fight *against* space, to affirm its own tempo there. That is great health, his combat with and against fatigue, the work of space-time in him. He says, *I auscultate myself with time, je m'ausculte avec le temps*.

The current neuro-bio-molecular and genetic model of the body finds a remarkable precursor in Michaux's work, a work centered on the feeling of the body's conscience, the blurring of formal borders, and a poetics of language where the sign is grasped in its materiality without excluding a strictly immanent lyricism. Medicine now replaces the traditional clinical work through the graphics of a complex imagery. It accentuates the parceling out, the pulverization of the body's representations in a formatted discourse saturated with acronyms that invade the natural languages. The body is, in its turn, at the same time an object of constant narcissistic concern and a building site of experimentation and artistic representation. Other forms of identity are about to appear more nuanced, perhaps, and refute strict dualisms.

In an important 1936 conference in Buenos Aires,[10] Michaux says that the role of the poet is to anticipate, to make a break, to bring something new (*to make breathable the unbreathable, habitable the uninhabitable, rendre respirable l'irrespirable, habitable l'inhabitable*) and to disappear, give way when the social norm catches up with him. If the air of the 'house of language' could become unbreathable and uninhabitable for a time, it can be a question of political circumstances like the war (*Ordeals, exorcisms, Epreuves, exorcismes,* 1940-1944), or simply of every-day language. J-M Rey writes, the language of the poet emerges from a body that *does not want to yield to the every-day nature of knowledge that is supposed to be contemporary to him, ne veut pas se plier à l'ordinaire des savoirs supposés lui être contemporains*. Hence, the example I quoted about *plasticity and flexibility* certainly would have been pointed to and distorted by Michaux in his own words and his laughter. It is thus, Rey adds,[11] that poetry testifies while fighting against *the most ordinary and the most aberrant effects of some of our knowledge, rebelling against the power of some of that knowledge, les effets les plus ordinaires et les plus aberrants de certains de nos savoirs, de se rebeller contre la puissance de certains de ces savoirs.*

Ironically, at present, the artists of the biotech or of genomic art have taken over certain of Michaux's graphics. They try to represent new forms and to grasp the mechanisms of living creatures in the process of making themselves, in the middle of the synthesis of proteins. Michaux, as a pioneer awakening the conscience through his writings, works for his health and for ours, for ours through his. He is also proof that the turning inward to oneself, the keen listening to one's body and the filtering of the world through one's own body does not prevent an accurate view of others, as his war poems testify.

In 1957, his friend Jules Supervielle[12] said of this visionary and studious poet, poète visionnaire et studieux, that he gave us : an anxious thirst, the nostalgia of thought. Indeed Michaux, this professor of unease, professeur d'inquiétitude, as J-P Martin[13] accurately calls him in his superb biography, always gives us something on to ponder. And it is also for this reason that he accompanies us.

Translation by Victor Hugo Velazquez

Notes

[1] B Edelman, *Nietzsche, un continent perdu*, PUF, Paris, 1999, p. 292-293.

[2] F Nietzsche, *Ecce Homo*, translation by W. Kaufmann, New York, 1967, p. 258: 'My formula for greatness in a human being is *amor fati*: that one wants nothing to be different, not forward, not backward, not in all eternity. Not merely bear what is necessary, still less conceal it – all idealism is mendaciousness in the face of what is necessary – but love it'; F. Nietzche, *Ecce Homo*, coll. 10/18, Paris, 1988, p. 59: ' *- la grandeur de l'homme s'exprime dans son* amor fati, *voilà ma formule ; ne pas demander de changement ni au passé, ni à l'avenir ni à l'éternité. Il ne faut pas se contenter de supporter ce qui est nécessaire, - il faut encore moins le cacher, tout idéalisme est mensonge face à la nécessité, - il faut l'aimer.* '

[3] Michaux, 'Bras cassé', Pléiade Vol. III, Gallimard, Paris, p. 855-886.

[4] C Malabou, *Que faire de notre cerveau?,* Bayard, Paris, 2004, p. 138-139.

[5] Michaux, 'My properties', *Selected Writings of Michaux*, translation by R Ellmann, New Directions Publishing Co., New York, 1968, p. 45.

[6] J-L Nancy, *L'intrus,* Galilée, Paris, 2000.

[7] Michaux, *Poteaux d'angle*, Paris, Gallimard, Pléiade, Vol. III, p. 1075. *Tent Posts*, translated by Lynn Hoggard, Green Integer, København, p. 137.

[8] ibid., p. 1061.

[9] *Chronicle of the pointsman/Chronique de l'aiguilleur*, Pléiade, vol. III, p. 14-15.

[10] Michaux, *L'avenir de la poésie*, Vol. I, Gallimard, Pléiade, Paris, p. 967-970.

[11] J-M Rey, 'Les paradoxes de la poésie', *Magazine littéraire*, N° 434, Paris, September 2004, p. 48-50 (volume dedicated to Artaud).

[12] Jules Supervielle, *Portrait de Michaux* (1957), Revue de La Bibliothèque Nationale, 14, Hiver 1984.

[13] Jean-Pierre Martin, *Henri Michaux*, Gallimard, Paris, 2004.

Bibliography

Danou, G., 'Henri Michaux et la médecine de soi'. Cerisy-La-Salle Conference, *Henri Michaux est-il seul?*, Les Cahiers bleus, Troyes, 2000.

Danou, G., 'Henri Michaux au cœur de la fatigue'. *Magazine Littéraire*, n° 411, July-August 2002.

Edelman, B., *Nietzsche un continent perdu*. PUF, Paris, 1999.

Malabou, C., *Que faire de notre cerveau?*. Bayard, Paris, 2004.

Martin, J-P., *Henri Michaux*. Gallimard, Paris, 2004.

Michaux, 'Bras cassé'. Pléiade Vol. III, Gallimard, Paris, 2004.

Michaux, 'My properties'. *Selected Writings of Michaux*, Translation by R Ellmann, New Directions Publishing Co., New York, 1990.

Michaux, *Poteaux d'angle*. Paris, Gallimard, Pléiade, Vol. III. *Tent Posts*. Translated by Lynn Hoggard, Green Integer, København, 1997.

Michaux, *L'avenir de la poésie*. Vol. I, Gallimard, Pléiade, Paris, 1998.

Nancy, J-L., *L'intrus*. Galilée, Paris, 2000.

Nietzsche, F., *Ecce Homo*. Translation by W Kaufmann, New York, 1967.

Rey J-M., 'Les paradoxes de la poésie'. *Magazine littéraire*, N° 434, Paris, September 2004.

Supervielle, J., *Portrait de Michaux*. Revue de La Bibliothèque Nationale, 14, Hiver 1984 (1957).

Tolstoy and the Making of the Inhuman

Knut Stene-Johansen

Abstract
Texts about illness and death may show how something unreasonable in a given literary text may be its own, profound reason. The illness' staging of a slow and escalating withdrawing of oneself, or, on the contrary, a fast and sudden end of life, teach us something about the fact that an ending can manifest itself long before the final, full point is set. This oscillation between life and death, where the unreasonable, accidental and causal unclear in the symptom's appearance become the only reason for the text, is well illustrated in Leo Tolstoj's short story 'The Death of Ivan Iljitsj'. When the actual illness is impossible to define, as more than just an illness, a specific problem arises concerning the very role of illness in human existence. *Ivan Iljitsj* is an example. The short story's subject is the 'material', inauthentic life of the bourgois. But it also deals with illness as a starting point for a change in the way of living, a change that breaks with the idea of death as only the death of 'Man' in a Heideggerian sense.

Key Words: Death; diagnosis; sickness in literature; Tolstoy

*****

> A free man thinks of nothing less than of death, and his wisdom is not a meditation upon death but upon life.
>
> Spinoza, *Ethics*, IV, proposition 67

Sickness in literature teaches us how sickness in life is also an interpretation of the world. When the sickness thematized in literature cannot be defined or clearly diagnosed, it provokes the question of the role of disease in human life. Leo Tolstoy's masterful short novel *The Death of Ivan Ilyich* offers an example of this. In a certain sense Tolstoy's goal seems to be to show how the inhumane is created, with sickness as the leading metaphor. Texts about sickness and death can also show how something unfounded in the text can be its foundation. Sickness's staging of a slow, gradual withdrawal from life, or on the contrary a quick and unexpected end to it, teaches us something of how an ending can manifest itself before a time is set for it. This exchange between life and death, where the baseless, random and causally uncertain in a set of symptoms become the text's only foundation, becomes evident in *The Death of Ivan Ilyich*, one of Russian literature's most famous novellas.

The story open with Ivan Ilyich's death and burial – more precisely with a report of Judge Ivan Ilyich's death – followed by a lengthy analepse leading up to that death. The news of Ivan Ilyich's death is received by his 'friends', including Piotr Ivanovich, who feels compelled to go to the memorial service. The widow is hypocritical, going around at the burial in a disturbed mix of authentic and inauthentic grief. Ivan Ilyich's story is 'the simplest, most ordinary and therefore most terrible', as it was. Ivan is described as a hypocritical striver, who certainly is fully taken up with his work. At the same time, he is also a Job, chosen for what seems to be a painful testing. And as Daniel Rancour-Laferriere and Gary R. Jahn among others has remarked, Ivan is also a Christ-like figure, suffering for sins other than his own. Initially and like another adventure figure, Ivan Ilyich goes to Petersburg to find a new job and by chance he gets one through a light form of corruption, employed by one of his 'friends'. Filled with enthusiasm he telegraphs his wife, he was 'completely happy'. The couple live and maintain their home as well-off people, but they lead a superficial life. Tolstoy is persuasive on this point: 'In reality it was just what is commonly seen in the houses of people who are not exactly wealthy but who want to look like wealthy people [...].' The life of Ivan Ilyich is filled with pettiness, climbing the ranks, bad moods and irritability. His job is described much like the medical profession.

The descriptions of Ivan Ilyich's life are thoroughly ironic. The furnishing of the new house in Petersburg, for example, is a showcase of unreality, which indeed might have a parallel in our contemporary design hysteria, with design that easily passes into self-parody. Ivan Ilyich manages to be so unlucky as to fall from a ladder. The fall, in which Ivan is struck in the side, constitutes an especially important episode in the story. The intermezzo is described with much understatment: 'The bruise was painful but it soon passed off'. As a matter of fact, it changes his life. Or at least, it may be interpreted that way, namely as a first sign of a coming catastrophe. The fall has been read as a biblical reference,[1] but it also has a comical element to it. Shortly after being thus upended while hanging some curtains, he must defend himself, and he tries to laugh at the episode:

> At tea that evening when Praskovya Fiodorovna among other things asked about his fall he laughed and showed them how he had gone flying and how he had frightened the upholsterer. 'It's a good thing I'm a bit of an athlete. Another man might have killed himself, whereas I got

> nothing worse than a knock here. It hurts if you touch it, but it's wearing off already – it's merely a bruise'.

He laughs about his fall, but what kind of laughter is it? Is it the philosopher's reflection and self-ironic chuckling? Evidently not. Ivan Ilyich's fall has probably nothing to do with illness as such, unless it has caused internal injuries, to the spleen, for example. But the blow does not seem at all so great that it could have caused such injuries. If that is the case, the fall becomes mainly symbolic, or readable as a symbol. As a parallel to the illness it will be able to lead to a recognition of thingliness, of being a thing subjected to the force of gravity. To perceive one's superficial existence is not the same as being cured of a lack of authenticity. 'To know inauthenticity is not the same as to be authentic,' wrote Paul de Man in 'The Rhetoric of Temporality'.

The fall takes place in the fourth chapter, with a crackling good opening: 'The whole family was in good health. Ivan Ilyich sometimes complained of a queer taste in his mouth and a sort of unconfortable feeling on the left side of the stomach, but one could hardly call that illness'. He consults a number of doctors and is quite irritable. His illness intensifies, and the intervals between become shorter and shorter. We witness a dynamic between marginalization of and focusing on the illness, with detailed descriptions of the pain. Ivan Ilyich says that he cannot identify with the general run of humanity, and he undergoes a quick negative evolution, concurrent with a further time compression: 'How it happened it is impossible to say because it came about step by step, imperceptibly.' Has the illness begun to live its own inside the narrative? Has it begun to problematize its own Hippocratic course, which goes so well with the narrative's beginning, middle and end? Or is it death that signals its arrival? Ivan Ilyich gets opium in any case, which progressively regresses him to childhood.

In a scene at that point in the novella, the strange person Gerassim holds Ivan Ilyich's leg on his shoulder. While in this most odd posture, Gerassim says: 'We shall all of us die, so what's a little trouble?'. In the end, in the tenth chapter, Ivan is totally isolated, yet in the center of his nearly Proustian redemption in memory. And so comes a change: for the worse, with bitter realizations. The doctor says that the moral pains are worse than the physical. The problem is that Ivan Ilyich realizes that he has not aimed high enough: 'Yet if only I could understand what it is all for. Even that's impossible. It might be explained if it could be said that I have not lived as I ought to have lived. But that could not possibly be said.' Then he dies, with a three-day-long shriek. The twelfth chapter is the story's shortest, with maximum intensity. Ivan Ilyich is 'redeemed' as death disappears and is replaced by light. He says: ''Death is over,' he said to himself. 'It is no more'.' Thus ends the novella. But Ivan Ilyich has indeed been dead from the first chapter onward. Tolstoy has played with the form, thus also with time, which gives the theme and key word 'death' an extra meaning: Death is always already there.

In a French edition, this text is included with two other novellas dealing with the theme of death in the most concrete sense, 'Three deaths' (1858) and 'Masters and servants' (1894). All three describe death through meetings with dead people – corpses, cold bodies – set before the living's gaze. The theme is quite well-known in Tolstoy, and explained by himself in the autobiographical *Childhood* (1852), *Boyhood* (1854) and *Youth* (1857), in the *Diaries* and in *A confession* from 1880. An early example of the theme is seen when, as a 24-year-old, Tolstoy writes of the first dead person he saw, namely his mother, who died when he was two years old, putting himself into the child's viewpoint:

> On a table in the middle of the room lay the coffin. Around it were candles that had burnt low in their tall silver candle sticks. In the far corner sat the chanter reading the Psalter in a low steady tone [...] The light, the gold brocade, the velvet, the tall candlesticks, the pink lace-trimmed pillow, the frontlet, the cup with ribbons, and something else of a transparent wax-like colour – all ran together in a strange blur. I climbed on to a chair to look at her face but there in its place I again saw the same pale-yellow translucent object [...] But why were the closed eyes so sunken? Why that dreadful pallor, and the blackish spot under the transparent skin on the cheek? Why was the expression of the whole face so stern and cold? Why were the lips so pale and their shape so beautiful, so majestic and expressive of such unearthly calm that a cold shiver ran over my spine and hair as I looked at them?

It is interesting to compare this passage from chapter 27 ('Grief') in Tolstoy's *Childhood* to the opening lines of Maxim Gorky's *Childhood* (1913). In both cases we find a child's eye for detail, which thus recalls, and tells us something about memory's often surprising proportions. This description illustrates the ungrounded in the text, the chance and apparent memory of small, insignificant details. Images that attach themselves to the child's retina become expressed in language two decades later by the 24 year-old writer. The experience has perhaps been gradually influenced by weaker impressions, and language becomes a method of saving the encounter with death from losing its existential significance. As Tolstoy scholar Geir Kjetsaa has remarked, death in Tolstoy appears as what Martin Heidegger in his 1927 magnum opus *Sein und Zeit* called 'life's existential phenomenon', and the story of the phony, lost and decayed Ivan Ilyich can perhaps be read as an illustration of Heidegger's distinction between authentic and inauthentic life. But it is not unproblematic to criticize Ivan Ilyich (or anyone else) for not perceiving that his being is not genuine, that he is an impersonal, inauthentic person, a 'yuppy'; even the deepest insight into inauthenticity lacks authenticity's guarantee. But it is literature, not philosophy that provides that insight. As in Hermann Hesse's *The Glass Bead Game*, it is clearer that all the most important rules of the game can be learned, but it requires an indirect kind of knowledge to master not just the game, but also its influence on the player.

Tolstoy was familiar with death. When he wrote Ivan Ilyich, his father, grandfather and two aunts who had each been his foster-mother had all died. In addition, he had seen death up close in the military. Later four of his children and a number of relatives and friends would die on him. Nor was suicide an unknown cause of death in his vicinity. His brothers Dimitri and Nikolas died in 1856 and 1860, with the latter's in particular having a strong impact. Tolstoy wrote in a letter to his brother Sergei on 24 September 1860 (Julian calendar) that death is the worst that can happen, and that 'When one says to oneself that it is the end of everything, it is basically no worse than life [...] the situation we find ourselves in is gruesome'.

An anxiety attack on the night of 3 September 1869, in which Tolstoy saw his own death, was a shattering experience that led to intellectual, philosophical and religious changes in Tolstoy. Ten years later he was in another crisis. He had in the meantime started a family, written *War and peace* and *Anna Karenina*, and devoted a lot of time to pedagogy. *The Death of Ivan Ilyich* was the first work written after his existential and spiritual crisis. But what is a crisis? Tolstoy endured many. It is perhaps first and foremost an outbreak of self-contempt, including contempt for the writing profession, and a violent clash with society, religion, country: a rejection of the whole world.

The story of Ivan Ilyich, written in 1884, thus initiates a new and final phase of Tolstoy's writing career. It was originally conceived as a first-person narrative in diary form. Presumably it was too difficult to have such a terminally ill character write a diary, and at the same time it seems as if Tolstoy wanted to take the pen away from Ivan.

The story's theme is bourgeois, material, inauthentic life. But it could also be said to be illness and fear of death as provoking an upheaval in life, such as can break down the rock-solid illusion that it is only 'people' who die. This naturally begs the question of how a theme like sickness and death can be introduced without the characters representing the theme losing credibility and becoming so deformed in their structural consistency that they tend to derail the reading rather than focus it on the theme.

The way of writing in the story is strongly marked by a kind of stylistic austerity or leanness with no place for picturesque or sensory descriptions or poetic turns. It is in a sense brutal, decidedly lacking in elegance, yet striving more toward symbolism than realism. Even in translation the sentences are complex, long and repetitive. Furthermore, the characters are described abstractly, with no richly detailed or image-saturated explanations. Everything points toward a theme that itself seems to take over or at least structure the form. Sickness narratives readily take on a 'Hippocratic' structure, with the traditional beginning, middle and end stages understood as symptom, diagnosis and outcome in the form of recovery or death. But as a supplement to this structure, which naturally includes back-sliding, uncertain periods, uneven steps toward recovery and placebo effects, a more textual, structured fusion is added, giving the story its spiral effect, with death in the center, and just at the narrative's actual arranged ending.

Repetition, non-chronological narration, everything points to sickness and death as the principle that both structures the narrative and rips apart the narrative form. Remaining within Russian literature, we need look no farther than the mentioned opening of Gorky's *Childhood*, where details in the child's experience of the father's death appear to be much more extraneous yet central to the writing style than the realistic, cold and merciless description of a black reality. Naturally the detail can be understood as a reality effect, but perhaps it is possible to see it as something more than a rhetorical necessity. Detail that overshadows the big picture can become a specific point for analysis. Detail dislocates the focus itself.

Tolstoy's story of Ivan Ilyich's illness and death is a good illustration of literary language's ability to handle the sickness theme. Tolstoy deploys his typical defamiliarizing or alienizing by, as mentioned, stripping the narrative of pictorial descriptions, interrupting the chronology and perhaps most of all by allowing the omniscient narrator to retreat in time to the advantage of the protagonist, who also gets the last word, be it only a death rattle. Tolstoy has otherwise used this technique of shedding light on reality or a character from a skewed perspective to the utmost in the novella 'Kholstomier', where life on a stud farm is described from a horse's point of view. But generally literary language operates in its deviation from normal language as able not only to capture the being of sickness, but also to be sickness' foremost spokesman.

When the story begins, with news of Judge Ilyich's death and the subsequent analepse, a narrative impairment is risked: a loss of suspense, nerve, tension, expectation. On the other hand, the text becomes more of a gloss, an 'explanation'. Analepses and everything that goes with them are readily more nuanced than film flashbacks, basically because reading a book is not the same as seeing a film. Here in Tolstoy it seems as if the first chapter's function is to open a privileged access to a main message that is not exhausted in the intrigue's culmination – the end that comes in the first chapter – but which is formed through Ilyich's afflictions until they end in visions and death.[2] By giving up uncertainty concerning the narrative's outcome, and thus renouncing suspense, Tolstoy avoids melodrama; he actually brings forth a drama. Tolstoy breaks with his adherence to the present form and what have been called his 'scenic' or 'panoramic' texts in this novella and deploys more a showing than a telling. For once he seizes on details from his character's past in order to hold life up to examination. For example, the medal Ivan receives when he takes his law exam bears the inscription *respice finem* – have regard for the end – and is significant to the reader in the sense that he precisely *cannot* do so. But for Ivan the inscription has a characteristic strategic meaning: he lives not just in the usual ignorance of his life's ending, but under the illusion that the end has no meaning.

At first the juridical milieu Ivan works in is described as completely cynical, inasmuch as the main preoccupations are who will succeed whom in the positions now available, and how far away from the center of town the burial will take place, how inconvenient it is to go to a funeral and how disturbing it is to have to offer condolences and go to the defunct's wake. Moreover, they all feel a bit glad: 'it is he who is dead, not I'. The lack of humanity, the very point of emphasis of the story, is quickly presented. For example, the first chapter describes Ivan Ilyich's closest friend, Piotr Ivanovitch, who must take on the duty of participating in the inquest and burial. His state of mind is one of desperation, he would rather play bridge, and leaves for a match right after the burial. It is he who is confronted with the late Ivan Ilyich. We quickly learn that conflicting diagnoses underlie the illness or are connected to Ivan's death. What is the diagnosis? Tolstoy would say he is sick in his soul. One of the doctors underscores this at the end, in a commentary which in its way opens for a critique of the excessive temporal authority exercised by the story's writer.

A translator's error sharpens the interpretive focus on this point. In one of the Norwegian translations, the pain is localized only to 'a stitch in the side' whereas the original states much more precisely the left side, that is, to the left of the stomach. The omission of such a detail is crucial to the diagnosis. For as soon as we know that it is on the left side individual and central organs can be excluded, as the liver and the appendix, while the left side is the heart's side. A symbolic dimension becomes more significant thanks to the precision the lacking translation led us to. More significant, to then disappear, one should say, since the medical exams that follow one another through the rest of the novella emphasize both the appendix and kidneys, among a number of other possible diagnoses. But the diagnosis is never made. Geir Kjetsaa describes the illness as stomach cancer, which does not seem implausible. However, as Gary R. Jahn also has remarked, the exact nature of Ivan's disease is perhaps beside the point. But as the illness receives no clear diagnosis in the course of the narrative, the novella becomes transparent, in Roland Barthes' sense of the word, that is, strong enough to tolerate significantly differing readings.

Illness is readily considered as pathology, understood as a type of abnormal condition. Medically speaking, pathology is the study of the body after death, a work of interpretation that turns out to be the most concrete dealing there is with death, and as a supplement to medical theory, furthermore, it constitutes a large field of medical history. Meanwhile, sickness is also normal. In the opening of Thomas Mann's *The Magic Mountain* doctor Krokowski says that he has never met a completely healthy person: 'Mir ist nämlich ein ganz gesunder Mensch noch nicht vorgekommen'. In this the schism between normal and abnormal another schism is formed, namely between the individual and the collective.

Are there situations in which one wishes to be sick? Evidently, but these are situations that are not unnaturally defined as asocial or pathological. It is not unusual for young men to attempt to evade military conscription via one or another feigned or exaggerated condition, or more dramatically, as in Henrik Ibsen's *Peer Gynt*, where the boy in the third act chops off a finger to avoid the King's service (to Peer's wonderment: 'To think it, wish it, even want it – but to do it! No, that I cannot understand!'). Self-inflicted injuries are known in religions (but also from youth psychiatry, extreme AIDS milieus, social services). But can one really desire illness? To wish oneself dead is to some extent intellectually comprehensible, if not acceptable, but to wish oneself sick? To wish oneself sick is in a sense not the opposite of wishing oneself healthy. To be sick is to find oneself in an undesired condition. But the condition of being sick is one that opens the way for a special recognition. Excessive health is also sick, as Adorno comments in *Minima Moralia*. Adorno says that there are those who are so obsessed with demonstrating their strength and vitality that one could take them for prepared corpses ['präparierte Leichen'], and that it is also death that lies behind that prevailing health ['Auf dem Grunde der herrschenden Gesundheit liegt der Tod'].

However, Adorno becomes just as moralistic as Tolstoy: the eternal life, to be lived as *das Man,* without consciousness of mankind's fate, without what Heidegger therefore calls 'being-unto-death' (Sein-zum-Tode). Ivan Ilyich lacks humility and love, and it is not until he is subjected to total suffering that his soul awakens. The relationship to his illness is marked by a lack of reconciliation. The pain, illness and suffering are characteristically enough called 'it', as G. W. Spence remarks.[3]

Not even the doctors, whether general practitioners or renowned specialists, can realistically counsel Ivan Ilyich: '[...] each of them said something different'. Their performance is described ironically, where they could just as well have represented a healthy rapport with the bodily. Tolstoy's scepticism about physicians is on a level with that found in Molière (for example in *The Imaginary Invalid, The Doctor Despite Himself* or *Dom Juan*). The doctors who appear in the novella are charlatans one and all, not because they act so hypocritically, but because they live on the same superficial level as lawyers or for that matter the entire entourage of the Golovin family, in brief, nearly everyone in the text. All the characters are functional. The wife is like a cardboard cutout, likewise the colleagues. We are dealing with Russian archetypes. The story's title points to this: Ivan Ilyich, not just 'Ivan', as with 'Gerassim', nor a formal Ivan Golovin, as in *Anna Karenina*, but something in between. The nearly exalted naïve Gerassim, the 'clean, fresh young peasant lad', he who holds Ivan Ilyich's leg on his shoulder, naturally has an especially clear function, but like the son Volodya, who has kept his feelings and openness, he does not belong to the ranks of superficial existences. As in Rousseau childhood is the point of departure for a critique of civilization. In addition to Rousseauian pantheism, there is a significant anticlericalism in Tolstoy.

It is in the sixth chapter that Ivan Ilyich articulates that he cannot identify with common humanity, and the so-called Caius syllogism ('Caius is a man, all men are mortal, therefore, Caius is mortal') is rejected by the sick judge. The passage underscores Tolstoy's message: We are all equal; Ivan Ilyich (and his death) shows how stupid it is to believe otherwise. Ivan protests that he is neither Caius nor common humanity, but a person completely different from all of the others. The Caius syllogism is a matter of the common versus the specific. The problem is that one cannot identify with part of a syllogism, or with the notion of the ego as a merely linguistic function. The notion that *das Man* dies, and not I, or rather that we live under the illusory belief that it is only 'one' – that is, no one – who dies, because 'one' is precisely no one, is trivial. For to turn it around, one can criticize Ivan Ilyich for not taking death to heart, but can *I*? Who am I to reproach others for not living in an authentic relationship to death? How can I know if I do so myself, even if I know what inauthenticity is? What choice is it that ensures a delusional relationship to death?

The novella reveals from all of its perspectives an irreconcilable lack of humanity, and tends toward becoming an exhibition of the literature of the inhumane. Tolstoy has also been criticized – by John Bayley, among others – for heavy-handedness in the desire to control a dying person's thoughts. Bayley writes in *Tolstoy and the Novel* that the death scene is too heavy and the forces deployed too authoritative. Undoubtedly there is a desire for control in this mode of writing. On the other hand there is a clear tendency toward a form of banalizing in the brief and intense text, which constantly unfolds like an attempt to take the individual out of play, to the benefit of a message about the fate of humanity. In this it is unlike *Anna Karenina*, where the same control over characters' thoughts is balanced by a sensitivity of the individual. It is the common run of humanity's inhumane side that is developed in the successful, ambiguous novel. Not even Ivan Ilyich's death is allowed to be individual.[4]

It all began with a condensed characterization of the bourgeois family and its apparent health. Behind the health, meanwhile, a latent illness lay hidden, a plague one could not be bothered about, because it did not fit into the materialistic model embraced by the upward-striving Russian bourgeoisie. When death so strongly dominates the novella, it may well be unbalanced. But the big question remains: How shall one *balance* death?

Translation by Thomas Petruso

Notes

[1] E Wasiolek, *Tolstoy's Major Fiction*, University of Chicago Press, Chicago, 1978, p. 173; and G R Jahn, *The Death of Ivan Ilyich. An Interpretation*, Twayne Publishers, New York 1993, p. 47.

[2] See C G Turner, 'The language of fiction: word clusters in Tolstoy's *The Death of Ivan Ilyich'*, in *MLR*, 65, 1970, p. 121.

[3] G W Spence, *Tolstoy the Ascetic*, Oliver & Boyd, London, 1967.

[4] J Bayley, *Tolstoy and the Novel*, University of Chicago Press, Chicago, 1966, pp. 214–215.

Bibliography

Adorno, T.W., *Minima Moralia. Reflexionen aus dem beschädigten Leben*, in *Gesammelte Werke*, bd. 4, Suhrkamp, Frankfurt am main, 1980 (1951)

Bayley, J., *Tolstoy and the Novel*. University of Chicago Press, Chicago, 1966.

De Man, P., 'The Rhetoric of Temporality', in *Blindness and Insight. Essays in the Rhetoric of Contemporary Criticism*,University of Minnesota Press, Minneapolis 1983.

Gorky, M., *Childhood*, Foreign Languages Publishing House, Moscow 1962.

Hesse, H., *The Glass Bead Game*, Owl Books, London 1980 (1943).

Jahn, G.R. *The Death of Ivan Ilyich. An Interpretation*, Twayne Publishers, New York 1993.

Rancour-Laferriere, D., 'Narcissism, Masochism and Denial in The Death of Ivan Ilyich', in: G.R. Jahn, *The Death of Ivan Ilyich. A Critical Companion*, Nortwestern U.P., Evanston, Illinois 1999.

Kjetsaa, G., *Lev Tolstoj. Den russiske jords store dikter*, Gyldendal, Oslo 1999; German trans., *Leo Tolstoj. Dichter und Religionsphilosoph*, Casimir katz Verlag, Gernsbach 2001.

Mann, T., *Der Zauberberg*, Fischer Taschenbuch verlag, 1998 (1924); eng. trans. *The Magic Mountain*, Everyman's Library, London 2005.

Spence, G. W., *Tolstoy the Ascetic*. Oliver & Boyd, London, 1967.

Tolstoy, L., 'The Death of Ivan Ilyich', in *The Death of Ivan Ilyich and Other Stories*, Penguin Classics, London 1960; *Childhood, Boyhood, Youth*, Penguin Classics, Harmondsworth 1985.

Turner, C.G., 'The Language of Fiction: Word Clusters in Tolstoy's *The Death of Ivan Ilyich'*. *MLR*, 65, 1970.

Wasiolek, E., *Tolstoy's Major Fiction*. University of Chicago Press, Chicago 1978.

III - ARCHEOLOGY

Treatment Politics:
The Rise of Radesyge Hospitals in Norway

Anne Kveim Lie

Abstract
This chapter discusses the rise of the radesyge hospitals in Norway. It will be argued that the end of the 18th century constitutes a historical moment where systematic treatment of patients in hospitals is formulated as a condition of possibility for the first time in Norwegian history. The radesyge hospitals are medicalized in a sense that the treatment intention permeates the whole institution in an unprecedented way in Norway. Nevertheless, focusing on their establishment as part of a teleological process towards the modern health care system obscures historical specificities, for instance the fact that medical experience was performed according to a totally different epistemology.

Key Words: History of medicine; radesyge

*****

In 1771, Collegium Medicum, the highest administrative organ in health affairs in Denmark-Norway, wrote in a letter to the head of the diocese in southern Norway that a disease called Radesyge was threatening the southern part of Norway.

> [It] is so dangerous, common, contagious and devastating to the entire population, and in particular to the army, that no measures would be too fast, effective or serious to stop and eradicate this confounded plague, before it gains so much ground, that the extensiveness either makes assistance impossible, or at least difficult or insufficient.[1]

In the letter, the Collegium Medicum was referring to several concerned reports they had received from local doctors as well as from the head of the diocese in Kristiansand, Hans Hagerup. Hagerup had pointed out that the disease increasingly spread out in his diocese, and that if no measures were taken more than the half of the population would be wrecked.[2]

What was this disease called radesyge? It is now largely forgotten, and hardly a word in the present Norwegian vocabulary. From about 1760 to about 1840, however, the disease was considered a major health problem in Norway. It was perceived as an important threat to society, not because it killed people, but because it 'destroyed' them. Originally, the concept Radesyge was probably a juxtaposition of the words *Rade* and *Syge*. *Syge* signified disease in Danish (sjuge in Norwegian), but the word *rade* was not a common word in contemporary Danish-Norwegian. The district surgeon Daniel Touscher told the Collegium Medicum, the highest administrative organ in health affairs, about the origin of the word in a letter from 1774:

> The word Rade has probably not been known for a long time, but the peasants have, especially in a few places in Lister county, embraced this word, fabricated in their own community, to describe a thing they consider harmful, evil or mean. For instance: a rada man, an evil man; a rada thing, a mean, harmful thing; a rada mare, a miserable, bad and obstinate mare, etc. Radesyge is, according to the peasant's understanding, a wicked and evil disease, which he, from its circumstances and consequences, considers a bad and almost untreatable disease.[3]

Hence in the beginning the word Radesyge probably signified an affliction that made ugly or evil. The patients suffering from Radesyge had deep ulcers on the whole body. The disease could also attack the mucous membranes and in advanced cases the skeleton, causing considerable deformities. Most authors describe an initial phase with catarrhalia, bone pains and light fevers.[4] The disease only gradually made its appearance, and often a great time span had elapsed before the victims became seriously ill. The nose and throat was frequently attacked, causing facial malformations and progressive difficulties in eating and drinking. According to most sources, untreated patients had to die a slow death, and walk around as 'living carcasses', a metaphor frequently used.[5] The nature of the disease remains unknown, although a series of articles has practiced the retrospective diagnosis of tertiary syphilis.[6] However, retrospective diagnosis remains a difficult genre,[7] and radesyge is an especially good example of this.[8]

Radesyge attracted considerable attention in the 100 years it haunted Norway. It was the subject of the first medical publications in a Norwegian setting,[9] and of the first dissertation ever at the new University of Christiania (present-day Oslo) in 1817.[10] The problem Radesyge was also met with a substantial amount of state initiatives. On the one hand, in this period a number of new medical officers were employed, largely to deal with this problem.[11] On the other hand, several so-called Radesyge-hospitals were founded, 16 in all, the first hospitals in Norway with a therapeutic intention.[12] Most of them later became the new municipality hospitals in the middle of the 19th century.

In this article, I will discuss the rise of the radesyge hospitals in the 1770s. The history of these hospitals has never been written, although in all reference works their constitution in passing is emphasized as one of the key events in Norwegian medical history.[13] In these accounts the radesyge hospitals are highlighted as important elements in the scientific development in Norwegian medical history, and as steps towards a more rational health care system in Norway. The historian Ole Moseng attributes the development of the Norwegian health care system in general and the hospital system in particular largely to the radesyge endemic, and claims that it was 'the modern hospital system which developed in Norway during the last decades of the 18th century'.[14] These hospitals are 'modern' according to Moseng primarily because for the first time treatment, and not care, was the prime objective of the stay in the hospital. He has, however, not conducted empirical studies of these hospitals. In what follows, I will explore the question of the development of the radesyge hospitals a bit further and ask: If these hospitals are so different, in what sense can they be said to be so? And in what sense may one talk of a curative intention in these hospitals?

1. Radesyge and Enlightenment Medical Politics: 'Incapable and Harmful Subjects'

Norway had by the time Collegium Medicum wrote their letter, only 5 officially appointed physicians, one in each diocese.[15] To that can be added about nine master and 25 journeymen surgeons, and five to six physicians in private practice, but in any case the country, which at that time was consisting of about 800 000 inhabitants,[16] was very sparsely covered with medical personnel.[17] The Norwegian peasantry had until then had little contact with medical authorities. In the diocese of Christiansand, there was only one officially appointed physician, and he seemed quite uninterested in visiting the rural areas.[18] The quacks dominated the medical marketplace in eighteenth century Norway.

Therefore it was not at all obvious that the radesyge problem had to be dealt with by the construction of hospitals, let alone extra doctors. Actually something rather extraordinary happened with the radesyge endemic, which probably was a combination of timing and the reported dramatic features of the disease. The latter half of the 18th century was definitely a period of increasing focus on disease as a problem demanding collective action.[19] The problem of the poor was included within the general issue of the health of populations, and charitable aid was largely replaced by a more general form of a 'medical police'.[20] The improvement of each body's utility now became an important factor in public health policy, and, at a state level, the physical health of the population was considered a relevant factor for economic management. That a health policy which regards the subjects' utility for the state of greatest relevance was prominent also in Denmark-Norway can be seen from the following statements from one of the members of the Collegium Medicum: 'A disease which creates so many incapable, even harmful subjects, cannot quickly enough be eradicated, and every parsimony that postpones the general treatment must be considered most harmful'.[21] The radesyge was regarded as incapacitating, chronic and contagious (although there was disagreement on this last point) and it was threatening to afflict an ever larger amount of the peasantry in the diocese, and ultimately Norway's inhabitants in general. Therefore, this disease was considered of importance also for the authorities in Copenhagen.

2. The Question of Hospitals in the International Debate

The late 18th century met with a new awareness of the utility of medical treatment. The question was not any longer whether medical treatment was useful, but how such treatment could best be administered. Should it be given at home or in special institutions? An extensive debate was conducted in European Journals and in several academic books. This debate is summarized in a voluminous article (470 words) under the headword *Kranken-Haus* in Krünitz' *Oeconomische Encyclopädie.*[22] The article defines hospital (Krankenhaus) as follows:

> Krankenhaus, das Haus, worin jemand krank liegt. In engerer und gewöhnlicher Bedeutung, ein öffentliches Haus, ein besonderes Gebäude, oder auch eine Anstalt, wo Kranke, insonderheit arme Kranke, verpfleget und curiret werden [...] Der Nahme Krankenhaus verdient im Deutschen vor allen gleichbedeutenden um deswillen den Vorzug, weil sein Begriff nicht so enge ist, als der von einem Lazareth, und nicht so vieldeutig wie der Ausdruck Hospital.[23]

What becomes clear from the extract of the contemporaneous debate concerning hospitals is that this is a historical moment where treatment of patients in hospitals is formulated as a condition of possibility for the first time in any breadth. On the one hand, there are strong arguments in favour of treatment in the patients' own home. There they could receive care from people who loved them and knew their needs. The commonest argument against hospitals is that they are too expensive. When treatment was ambulatory, the patients paid their own diet and housing, and they were spared of the long and hazardious travel to the hospital. They could also continue their occupation as far as possible, which kept them in the production.

However, the majority of the authors preferred the hospital as the best solution for several reasons. The Danish doctor Johann Gabriel Hensler, admitted in his thesis *Ueber Kranken-Anstalten* that ambulatory treatment had its advantages. Absolute prerequisites for a successful cure was that the patients received their medication at right intervals and in correct amounts, that they were provided with healthy, nutritious and fresh food, and that they were taken care of in clean, light and airy surroundings. The problem with ambulatory treatment was that most patients were poor, which meant that all these prerequisites had to be prejudiced in some way or another. For this part of the population treatment in hospitals was absolutely unavailable, Hensler thought.[24]

In the *Birth of the Clinic* Michel Foucault argued that hospitals were irrelevant to medicine before the founding of the medical clinic, mainly due to epistemological reasons. The disease could for the 18th century doctor, according to Foucault, only be grasped in its local, natural locus, the patients' home:'Like civilization, the hospital is an artificial locus in which the transplanted disease runs the risk of losing its essential identity'.[25] However, in this large debate reflected in the 450 page long article in Krünitz, epistemological arguments are not put forward at all, this is a far more pragmatic discussion. The questions are: Where could treatment best take place, how can we rehabilitate the patients as rapid as possible back to society? Michel Foucault also argued that the thought of an individualized treatment made the thought of hospitals impossible.[26] Here, in the international debate, it is the other way around. Precisely the need for individualized treatment, that every treatment has to be tailored according to the patients constitution, is put forward as an argument for hospitals. Individualized treatment presupposed not only that the patients took their individually prescribed medications, it also demanded a meticulous diet which the poor were unable to handle. In their local communities the patients also engaged in practices which the doctors found most damaging to the tailored treatment. Not only did they often demand bloodletting uncritically from the local practitioner, they also involved with quacks, who gave the same treatment to everybody regardless of the individualized conditions.

To conclude, the foundation of the first hospitals with a curative intention in Norway takes place in an international context where the question is extensively debated. However, what makes the Norwegian context special is that these hospitals are founded as result of the radesyge endemic.

3. A New Era: The Radesyge Hospitals

By rescript of 22. of April 1772 it was decided that three surgeons should travel around in the county of Stavanger, in the west coast of Norway, to offer treatment. An organization of a domestic form of hospitalization lied at the base of these new incentives. At places where it was considered necessary, the surgeons should establish small temporary wards that could be abandoned when they had filled their functions. Medicaments should be distributed freely, under the authority of the doctors designated by the authorities. In the same rescript, a hospital in Stavanger was also planned for persons 'who have the so-called Radesyge in an advanced stage, with *carie ossium* etc'.[27] This city hospital was modelled on the older almshouses, as a place for caring, and was not intended to be a curing place (the cure should take place in the temporary wards).

However, the surgeons reported several difficulties in fulfilling their order. Complicated transportation made transfer of doctors and food almost impossible. Houses could not be rent for the temporary wards. The doctors claimed that the amount of patients possible to treat at the same time under these circumstances was very limited, whereas in a permanent hospital they would be able to treat at least 25 at a time. It was also argued that the peasants' bad living habits complicated the cure. Their 'bad habits' were contrary to the order, cleanliness and a healthy diet, all of which were absolutely indispensable if a fortunate cure was to be obtained. A permanent hospital could save money, they finally argued. The lousy diet in the private houses drastically reduced the efficiency of the medication, with the effect that more medicines than what under ideal circumstances in a hospital was necessary had to be spent.[28] We here easily recognize the arguments from the international debate referred to earlier.

In a rescript from June 1773, the wording was changed. There were still plans for a hospital in Stavanger (due to several reasons the other had not yet been built). However, this time it was not intended as a caring institution for the most affected persons, on the contrary treatment was the main purpose. It was explicitly stated that incurable should not be admitted. The county governor in Bratsberg suggested that men and women in their fertile age should be given priority, and that no clergymen should consecrate a couple without a health certificate.[29] The treatment should thus be provided for those persons who could be strengthening the power of the state, and as such it emerges as one of the central issues of mercantilist politics. In October 1773 a hospital for Radesyge opened in Stavanger.[30] The next four years, three other hospitals for Radesyge only were established in Norway, one in Flekkefjord (1775), a smaller one in Mandal (1776), and the biggest in the east part of the diocese, in Bratsberg, near present day town Skien (1774).[31] Each of them was small, having only 20 to 40 beds.

4. The Radesyge Hospitals as Arenas for the Production of Experience

It has been argued that these hospitals are early versions of the medical clinic.[32] Towards the end of the eighteenth century hospitals had begun to attain a privileged position regarding knowledge production. Medical knowledge was increasingly regarded as something that could only be gained through experience, also in Denmark-Norway. However, not all experiences carried equal weight: As can be seen from the name given to the quacks, empirico or empiric, the question of experience was a problematic one.[33] The experience of the empirics, or quacks, had to be contrasted with scientific observation in order to preserve the physicians' authority. The empiric collected data simply and casually, whereas scientific observation was supposed to be a kind of reasoned empiricism that could only be done by the physician. Until the last half of the eighteenth century there was no consensus as to where this kind of experience was to take place. The famous Boissier de Sauvage had been collecting his experiences out in the field, in the homes of private clienteles, in the hospital ward, in the dissection theatre, in the nursery, or in his own family.[34] In a lot of European countries there was, however, in the latter half of the eighteenth century, an attempt to privilege the hospital as a particular locale for observation. Teaching hospitals were established in Vienna, in London and Edinburgh, to name a few. It was generally acknowledged that what was needed was a multiplicity of experiences, and that the hospital was the best place to obtain these experiences. The hospitals, according to the new experiential paradigm, provided better possibilities for thorough observation – patients were lined up in beds, they could be compared, and followed through a longer period of time. Other environments in which patient and practitioner met, it was argued, were too unstable. The hospital was also an ideal institution for maintaining the distinction between the learned practitioner and the empiric. It stabilized the physician's status in the empiricist environment and gave credit to empirical knowledge as something else than the empirics' random practice.[35]

Also in the Danish-Norwegian context increasing attention was focused on the hospital as a place for the accumulation of knowledge-gaining experience towards the end of the century. The first teaching hospital, a general hospital, was established in Copenhagen in 1757, and hospital instructions stated that the physician should teach medical students.[36] The value given to observation in the hospital was increasingly stressed, and its chief physician Frederik Ludvig Bang published his elaborate hospital diary in 1789, based on observations in the hospital.[37]

Radesyge was new to the medical world, it was not known to anybody but to the peasants who suffered from it. Their doctors' obligation to report observations concerning disease symptoms, treatment, and treatment outcome is stated already in the first instruction to the surgeons leaving for Norway in 1772.[38] The instruction was in fact called a *preliminary* instruction (*Interims Instruction*), and the reason for the preliminary character was that it was considered revisable according to experience obtained at places where the disease was ravaging. One of the main reasons given in the resolutions for the construction of the hospitals was in fact the need for a collection of observations regarding the disease. The formal instruction to the hospital doctors explicitly stated their duty not only to keep clinical records but also to send these records to Copenhagen regularly, together with the accounts. In fact, several times the authorities demanded more observations, more facts about symptoms, treatment outcomes etc.[39] The therapeutic efficiency had to be combined with medical knowledge. Or rather, the optimal therapeutics presupposed the construction of proper knowledge, the gathering of the maximum amount of observations regarding radesyge.

How then was knowledge in these hospitals produced? It is evident from the hospital journals and the quarterly reports sent to the Collegium Medicum, that the empirical observations about the disease and its cure are not facts to be accounted for by complex causal narratives about qualitative, chemical, or mechanical changes to the body's solids and fluids. On the other hand, neither is the medical observer searching for organ localization or pathological changes: Not in a single case do they report autopsy findings. Rather, they are focusing on the surface of the body, meticulously searching for similarities and differences. These texts never discuss differential diagnostics. The facts they are establishing tell us how they observed and what they observed, as well as what they did not care to look for. The patient records indirectly display a conception of the body as a system in balance and in balance with its surroundings. The constitutions of individuals and of places are highlighted in terms of qualities such as hot and cold, wet or dry. Often the radesyge patients are reported to have a 'cacochymical constitution'.[40] The ulcers are described in a qualitative manner, using words as 'deep', 'large', 'with a strong stench', and with elaborate descriptions of color nuances. Radesyge was obviously considered a constitutional disturbance, to be rectified by changes of regimen or of place, by medicines to raise or depress, by bleeding, by warmth or cold, feeding or starving, vomiting or purging etc, in addition to the more specific treatment of mercury. The texts written by the hospital doctors provide discriminations which depend on knowing individual biographies, constitutions and circumstances. The question of the cause of the disease is almost absent; it is the symptomatic outcome that matters. In this connection, the question of contagion, as a special variant of the question of cause, seems quite irrelevant. It is not that they do not mention it, it is rather that the question of contagion does not seem to bring about any fundamental changes in the conclusions neither regarding the nature of the disease nor regarding treatment regimes. When the question is posed, it is stated in moral terms, transforming the discourse from a purely descriptive one to a moral one. An example could be cited from the journal of dr. Steffens in Stavanger, describing one of his patients:

> Da er aber ein grosser Freund aller Unordnung war, so lief er 2 Mahl aus den Kranken-Hause, und da sein Übel einzig und allein seiner Lebens Arth zugeschrieben wurde, und es ohnedem zu befürchten war, dass er sich bald nachdem er völlig geheilt seyn würde dieses Übel wieder durch seyn unordentliches und faules Leben zuziehen würde, hielt man es vor überflüssig ihm von neuen mit gewalt hieher bringen zu lassen.[41]

Contagion is here an element justifying the decision not to treat the patient further; it simply is not worth it. It is not at all a question of bringing the patient back to treatment in order to prevent more people from being infected. Accordingly, contagion is not affecting the treatment policy, it affects the moral verdict.

The hospital records and reports constitute, thus, a discourse where the rendering of nature, notation of observations as they appear to the doctors' gaze, is the important element. Philosophical judgments regarding the nature or cause of the disease are in fact seldom performed, and if they are, it is as a result of direct questioning from Copenhagen. The function of these hospitals was obviously not to establish new scientific knowledge on the spot, they can rather be said to constitute premise suppliers, in the form of experience as raw material, for the central medical consciousness in Copenhagen.

5. 'The Surest Means to Cure'

The most important intention with these new hospitals were, however, not the collection of experience, but the treatment of Norway's diseased inhabitants. In the introductory correspondence to the founding of the hospital in Flekkefjord, it was stated by Collegium Medicum that they had always regarded 'the foundation of hospitals as the surest means to this dangerous disease's complete and absolute cure, because the ambulatory way of curing is slow and insufficient'.[42] Treatment was the main aim of these hospitals, a fact which is stated in several letters from the King and also in the hospitals' foundation papers. These institutions were never referred to as places for care and nursing. The radesyge patients were admitted to the hospital for treatment and isolation during a limited amount of time. The hospitals were not supposed to admit untreatable patients, and several times the doctors were reminded that the maximum stay should not exceed six months.[43]

What kind of treatment was offered in these hospitals? Firstly, there was a considerable variation. Attention to age, sex, temperament and habit was essential for assessing each person's constitution and predicting how the individual patient would sustain the effects of disease as well as therapy. The hospital surgeons pointed out that within general guidelines treatment had to be carefully tailored to each personal case, and this assured a wide therapeutic arsenal. The therapeutic agents were given with the expectation that they would produce systemic changes and thus carry off the disease. By diarrhea, salivation, vomiting, bloodletting or with evacuation of pus from the wounds, it was thought that the disease would leave the body.

Henrik Steffens in Stavanger distinguished between *mundificantia* and *laxatives*, medicaments which performed functions on blood and the digestive system, respectively ('die gewöhnliche zur verbesserung ihrer Säfte dienlichen Mittel'). *Laxatives* should be used on a weekly bases, and they were supposed to bring about the evacuation of the disease-causing stools. Jalap (a resinous cathartic plant from Mexico), and medicinal rhubarb were the most commonly used laxatives. The *mundificantia*, or blood cleansing medicines, were used twice a day, more if the patient was considered strong enough.[44] Steffens prepared a *Decoctum mundificatium* that was a mixture of grass, dandelion root, guajac tree and pine cones.[45] Almost all patients were also given antiscorbutic medication, mainly *trefoil*, *scurvy grass* or *China root*.[46] In most cases the radesyge doctors would give *mercury*, but only after the antiscorbutic cure was finished, because they held that scorbutic patients did not tolerate mercury.[47] The physician in the hospital in Flekkefjord, Henrik Deegen, normally gave *sublimate mercury*, as pills, the so-called internal cure. Steffens normally applied mercury in the form of unction, or the external cure. Occasionally he also prescribed *Mercurium Dulcium*, or sweet mercury, as powder for internal administration. Both used mercury in order to obtain salivation, and considered salivation the main aim of the treatment, but stressed that it had to be moderate, in order to avoid serious side-effects. However, they also both emphasized that if there were obvious signs of venereal disease (that is, genital wounds or *fluore alba* (discharge) the salivation should be more powerful, whereas without such signs it should always be mild. They also performed surgical interventions, such as bloodletting, and the application of *vesicatories* in order to obtain blisters so that the disease matter could be let out. The wounds were dressed with *digestives*, and *fomentations* of hot water were frequently applied in order to make the blood accumulate at the wounded area and release the pathological matter. Steffens was also applying '*Fontanellen*', or artificial ulcers for the discharge of bad humours. Another frequently used medicament was *Laudanum Liquidum Sydenhami*, or drops consisting of opium, cinnamon, cloves and saffron, used as an analgesic and hypnotic. A few times Steffens also notes the use of a medicine called *Theriaca Andromachi*, a compound of 64 elements, one of them being snake flesh, reduced by means of honey to an electuary. This medicine had its origin in antiquity, and was originally a kind of antidote to snake poison, but became more and more of a panacea from the Middle Ages on.[48] *Antimonium* is a medicament used by all the hospital doctors, either as a *mundificative* or as a *diaphoretic*, usually in the form of powdered antimony ore, *Antimonium Crudum*.

These were the most important medical remedies administered in the radesyge hospitals, but the list is far from complete. To show that medication was in fact given, is, however, not sufficient to state that the radesyge hospitals were fundamentally different from the earlier types of institutions. In fact, already in the 16th century in the German Blatter Haus, medical treatment was considered an important aim of the institution, and medication was frequently given.[49] In Norway, several trials were conducted sporadically in the leprosy hospitals by interested physicians.[50] It is thus not correct to argue that the fact that treatment is given in itself make the radesyge hospitals special in Norwegian medical history. In the next chapter I will focus on what in my opinion constitutes the fundamental change in these institutions vis-à-vis the older institutions. The main difference between these new hospitals and the earlier ones, is not the fact that medication was administered per se, rather that the treatment intention permeates the whole institution, in such a way that it gives sense to talk of a medicalized institution.

6. The Radesyge Hospitals as Medical Arenas

We have seen that curing was the prime aim of these institutions. This intention is reflected already from the beginning. In the rescript which directs the foundation of the hospital in Stavanger, it was stated that the treatment should be granted by the surgeons Henrik Steffens and Johannes Christian Tychsen, who were supposed to be there full time. Thus, the intention of treatment was fundamental in these hospitals. How was this reflected in the shaping of the hospitals and in the hospitals' practice? I hope it will be clear in what follows, that these new institutions were medical arenas in a way that the older institutions never were. Everything from the architecture of the hospitals to the patients' diet regimes and the cleaning of the building was subject to medical regulations. First and foremost this is the case with the doctor's role as the initiator and incontestable authority in these new institutions. For the first time in Norway, the uninterrupted presence and hierarchical privilege of the doctor was established in hospitals. The hospital in Stavanger had two full-time doctors present. Salaries to the physicians were supposed to stimulate treatment efficiency. The physician in Bratsberg got eight Riksdaler for each patient, and only the half for those who died, and nothing for the treatment of relapsed patients (which was nevertheless his duty).

A closer look at one of the instructions for hospital construction, Bratsberg, reveals that the doctor was also given priority in forming the therapeutic environments. The original rescript is extraordinarily detailed. The local physician, Johannes Møller, who had been appointed regional physician (landphysicus) in Bratsberg in 1773 (rescript of 6.10 1773), had made the drafts. Here he proposed the establishment of a hospital based on treatment, because 'in Bratsberg county the in several parts of Norway rampanting so-called Radesyge is expressing itself increasingly'.[51] And the object is clearly stated: 'It is necessary', the rescript continues, 'in order to see the people burdened with this disease cured, that a hospital in this county is erected'.[52] The intention is materialized in the hospital's architecture: The interior specified in these instructions is no longer one of assistance, but of therapeutic action; the internal space was organized in order to make it medically efficacious. All the factors which made the hospital dangerous for its occupants had to be excluded. The problem of dirt, of stagnant and miasmatic air, and of the hospital as disease-breeding place had to be confronted by an architecture that minimized these kinds of problems.

The house was to be placed in 'the healthiest and most convenient place'.[53] The building proposed should have four patient rooms, each with ten beds, separated from the kitchen by a hallway. Patient rooms should not be located in direct communication with food preparing facilities. The patient rooms were further separated according to different functions; two of the rooms were reserved for the people most affected or in the strongest cure, one for each gender. The other two rooms were reserved for less affected and convalescent patients. The lavatory was kept out of the hospital area; in fact there were two lavatory buildings, one for the sick and one for the healthy. There were windows in each room, to allow for enough light. The focus on therapy can further be seen from the specification not only of a special room for medicaments only, but also for a room 'at the doctor's service',[54] where inspections could take place. The instruments for the preparation of medicaments are also specified; stone pots to prepare decocts, jars to preserve them, special spoons (of tin, not of wood) and cups for medication intake.

The doctor had a considerable influence in the hospitals' daily life. The 'oeconomicus' was supposed to 'promote the cleanliness of the hospital', but the cleaning should take place according to the physicians' request.[55] The oeconomicus should clean the beds regularly by airing and fumigation, and he was also responsible for the 'washing of sheets and patients',[56] as well as changing straw in the rag sacks in the beds when asked to do so by the doctor. Food and drink was also the responsibility of the oeconomicus, but it was stressed again that this should happen only 'after the doctor's orders', and 'in accordance with his treatment regimes'.[57] A housekeeper (oppvarterske) was supposed to 'supervise the sick, so that they do not get something that I [the doctor] do not allow'.[58]

In a contract signed between the oeconomicus and the doctor in Flekkefjord sygehus the food and meal regularities are prescribed. The meals were supposed to be provided at exact times: breakfast at 8.30 am, dinner at 11, and supper at 6.30 pm – 'sharp', the surgeon stresses. Order was of uttermost importance, and was considered vital not only as a disciplining factor, but also certainly as a means of treatment; disorder could disturb the entire treatment process. Regarding the prescribed food in this contract, which is more or less the same in the meal lists that exist for all the radesyge hospitals, two things are noteworthy: Firstly, it did not contain any fish, although these hospitals were situated at the coast, where fish would be the most common food. If the peasants at the countryside would at all eat meat, they would eat it salted or dried,[59] whereas the food provided in the hospital was fresh meat soup, oatsoup or barley soup. This made sense according to early modern medical diet preferences,[60] but certainly not according to practical arrangements. Diet was used as a medical technology, as a means of treatment to the patients.

We see that during these years hospitalization became the basis, and also on several occasions, the condition, for a therapeutic approach. The instructions regarding therapy ensured a relatively fixed amount of therapeutic measures. The hospitals thus tended towards becoming essential elements in medical technology, not simply as places for curing, but as instruments which made curing possible (due to disorder in the way of living among the poor). People considered untreatable should not be admitted, and the time spent in the hospital should not exceed six months.[61]

These hospitals were supposed to be 'curing machines', to borrow an expression from Jaques Tenon: as institutions in which medical science was perfected and in which cures were systematically achieved.[62] Treatment had replaced caring as the principal aim of the hospital, and that is reflected in everything from treatment procedures to the hospitals' interior. These hospitals as treatment institutions are not unique in an international setting; similar developments took place in a number of European cities at the time.[63]

7. Conclusion

On what ground can these hospitals be called groundbreaking events in Norwegian medical history? And more specifically: On what levels can we speak of a discontinuity here? When it is argued that the radesyge hospitals represent the growth of the 'modern health care system', it is difficult to agree. That is first and foremost due to the word 'modern', which is at the best vague and imprecise. These hospitals are certainly not modern in the sense that they are the equivalent of the clinics of the 18th century. To qualify these hospitals by virtue of later institutions, makes it easy to overlook their historical specificities. The radesyge hospitals are small, they are intended for one disease only, and the medical experience gathered here belongs performed here there is no systematic comparison of patients.

Traditionally, the rise of the hospitals as 'curing machines' has been linked to fundamental epistemological shifts. A recent work on Norwegian medical history in the early modern period has emphasized the combination of a new structural reorganization with a new 'analytical tool' in the late eighteenth century. The same author also describes this period as undergoing a gradual 'transition away from tradition and imitation of the ancients towards experience and experiments'.[64] This has also repeatedly been argued in the historiography of the radesyge.[65] However, we have seen that the way experience was produced in these hospitals was very different from what medical experience came to be in the 19th century. The experience gathered in the radesyge hospitals implied a different conceptual and epistemological world, a world where other objects were relevant to the medical observation than what was the case 100 years later. As Ludwik Fleck observed, 'direct perception of form (Gestaltsehen) requires being experienced in the relevant field of thought'.[66] That is to say, there is no 'pure' experience, it all depends on how you look and what you look for. The doctors definitely observed in these hospitals, but according to a fundamentally different epistemology.

That being said, it is obvious that the radesyge hospitals did represent a fundamental discontinuity on an institutional level. For the first time in Norwegian history, the hospitals were designed as places for treatment, not for caring. As we have seen, medical treatment was administered in the old type of institutions also. But compared to the earlier hospitals, the radesyge hospitals constitute a more differentiated and medicalized facility. This is partly because the doctor plays such a central part in initiating, planning and running the hospitals. As important is, however, that the entire practice and functioning of these hospitals is directed towards the promotion of medical treatment. The architecture is supposed to fulfill medical functions, the cleaning shall take place according to medical demands, and the feeding of the patients is determined by medical considerations. This, in my opinion, makes it fruitful to refer to the rise of the radesyge hospitals as a qualitatively new phenomenon in Norwegian medical history.

Notes

[1] Letter from Collegium Medicum to Hans Hagerup 17.9.1771 'er saa farlig, almindelig, smittsom, og ødeleggende paa det heele Folke-Færd, og in Specil paa Land-Militien, at der ikke kan tages hastige, virksomome, og alvorlige Foranstaltninger nok til at standse og udrydde denne ælendige Lande-Plage, førend den faaer grebet saa vidt om sig, at Vidtløftigheden giör enten Hielpen ugiörlig, eller i det mindste heel vanskelig og ufuldkommen. In: The National Archive in Oslo, Cabinet nr 9 (Radesykeskapet), Package 165 A-C. (All references to this package will in the following be referred to as RA).

[2] See letter from Hagerup to Collegium Medicum 15.12.1769: 'der har paa nogle Aar begyndt at grassere en landsfordærvelig, saltflodagtig og anstikkende Sygdom blant Almuerne her i Stiftet, som man her til Lands har givet Navn af Radesyge [...] den æder alt mer og mer om sig, saa at hvis derpaa ei strax raades Bod, saa ødelægges mer end den halve Deel af Indbyggerne.' For the other reports, see e.g. letters from Adam Cron, physician in the diocese of Kristiansand Febr. 1770 and 17.9.1771, RA.

[3] 'Det Ord, Rade, er vel ikke noget egentlig gammelt eller længe siden bekiendt Ord, men Bonden har i sær paa nogle steder i Lister Amt, antaget dette af dem selv opdigtede Ord, til at betegne en Ting som de anseer for skadelig, slem og ond, ex en rada Mand, en skarnsagtig, ond Mand, en rada Ting, en slem, skadelig Ting, en rada Mærr, en usel, slet og Tradsig Mærr, etc. Radesygen er altsaa i Bondens Forstaaelse, en slem og ond Sygdom, som han anseer af dens Omstændigheder og Følgerne, for en slem og næsten ulægelig Sygdom'. D. Touschen , Stavanger 6 Mars 1774. In: RA (as in footnote 1)

[4] See for instance Christian Elovius Mangor, *Underretning om Radesygens Kiendetegn, Aarsager og Helbredelse* (Kiøbenhavn: Johan Frederik Schultz, 1793). or Henrik Deegen, *Noget om Radesygen, observeret ved Sygehuuset i Flechefiord og udgivet til Nytte for Almuen* (Christiansand:

Andreas Swane, 1788). For a later summary se for instance Friedrich Ludwig Hünefeld, *Die Radesyge, oder Das skandinavische Syphiloid: aus skandinavischen Quellen dargestellt* (Leipzig: L. Voss, 1828).

5 '[D]e see ud som levende Aadseler, og snige sig omkring som Skrækkebilleder for sine Medmennesker' Rasmus Frankenau, *Det offentlige Sundhedspolitie under en oplyst Regiering: især med Hensyn paa de danske Stater og deres Hovedstad: en Haandbog for Øvrigheder og Borgere* (København: Poulsen, 1801), p. 78.

6 This practice started with Carl Wilhelm Boeck: 'Klinik over Hudsygdommene og de syphilitiske Sygdomme'. In: Norsk Magazin for Lægevidenskaben 6 (1852), 273-330. Other examples are C.J. Borge, 'Radesygen,' *Tidsskrift for den norske lægeforening* 25, no. 12 og 13 (1905): 427-32, 67-75, and Jens Henrichs: 'Kan Radesygen tillægges nogen betydning i vore sindslidelsers ætiologi?' In: Norsk Magazin for Lægevidenskaben 74 (1913), 881-916.

7 Jon Arrizabalaga, 'Syphilis,' i Kenneth F Kiple (red.), *The Cambridge World History of Human Disease*, (Cambridge: Cambridge University Press, 1993), p. 1029.

8 Anne Kveim Lie, 'Tanker om radesyken i Norge – 'den hentærer sine Offere langsomt',' *Tidsskrift for den norske lægeforening* 123, no. 24 (2003): 3562-4. Anne Kveim Lie, 'Radesykens tilblivelse' (Phd. thesis, University of Oslo, 2008), esp. Ch. 1.

9 Deegen, *Noget om Radesygen.*

10 Fredrik Holst: *Morbus Quem Radesyge vocant*. Christiania 1817.

11 The amount of officially appointed civilian medical officers (physicians and surgeons) physicians grew considerably, from about 10 around 1750, to 47 in 1814. John Utheim, *Oversigt over det norske civile Lægevæsens historiske Udvikling og nuværende Ordning, Bilag 2 til den kongelige Lægekommissions Indstilling.* (Oslo: Johannes Bjørnstads Bogtrykkeri, 1901).

12 See for instance Frederik Holst, 'Sygehuse for venerisk Syge, Radesyge og andre ondartede Hudsygdomme i Norge i Decenniet fra 1822 til 1831,' *Eyr* 10 (1834): 1-44. The actual number depends on whether one includes the hospitals for venereal disease. See also Ole Georg Moseng, *Ansvaret for*

undersåttenes helse 1603-1850, bd. 1 i *Det offentlige helsevesen i Norge 1603-2003*, (Oslo: Universitetsforlaget, 2003)., pp 235-71.

[13] See for instance I. Reichborn-Kjennerud, I. Kobro og Fredrik Grøn, *Medisinens historie i Norge* (Oslo: Kildeforlaget, 1985).

[14] Moseng, *Ansvaret for undersåttenes helse 1603-1850*, p. 235.

[15] Actually, only one of them was responsible for a diocese, the other four had their responsibility to the towns of Bergen, Christiania, Trondheim and Kongsberg.

[16] Statistisk sentralbyrå, *Historisk statistikk 1968*, *Norges offisielle statistikk* (Oslo: Statistisk sentralbyrå, 1969), p. 44.

[17] Utheim, *Oversigt over det norske civile Lægevæsens historiske Udvikling og nuværende Ordning*, p. 7.

[18] See for instance rescript 28.4 1748 in L. Thurmann, *Samling af Love, Forordninger, kongelige Rescripter og Resolutioner, Placater, Reglementer, Instruxer, Fundatser og andre offentlige Aktstykker vedkommende Læger, Apothekere, Dyrlæger og Gjordemødre i Kongeriget Norge* (Christiania: 1851), p. 16.

[19] Johann Peter Frank, *System einer vollständigen medicinischen Polizey*, 2 utg. (Mannheim: Schwan, 1784); Frankenau, *Det offentlige Sundhedspolitie*. See also Michel Foucault, 'The Politics of Health in the Eighteenth Century,' i Colin Gordon (red.), *Power/Knowledge: Selected Interviews and Other Writings 1972-1977 By Michel Foucault*, (New York: Pantheon Books, 1980).

[20] Foucault, 'The Politics of Health in the Eighteenth Century.'

[21] 'Da en Sygdom, som giør saa mange uduelige, ja skadlige Undersåtter, ikke gesvindt nok kan blive udryddet, og maa enhver Sparsommelighed, som altmer opholder den almindelige Cuur, ansees for høyst skadelig' Letter from Collegium medicum to head of Stavanger county Scheel 29.9 1774. RA (as in footnote 1).

[22] Johann Georg Krünitz, *Oeconomische Encyklopädie, oder allgemeines System der Staats-Stadt- Haus- und Landwirthschaft in alphabetischer Ordnung*, 242 bind (Berlin: Pauli, 1773-1858), vol. 47 [1789], pp. 121-590.

[23] Ibid., vol. 47 [1789], p. 120.

[24] Philipp Gabriel Hensler, *Ueber Kranken-Anstalten* (Hamburg: 1785). Sitert fra utdrag av samme i Krünitz; Krünitz, *Oeconomische Encyklopädie*, vol. 47 [1789], pp. 121-145.

[25] Michel Foucault, *The Birth of the Clinic: An Archaeology of Medical Perception* (London: Tavistock, 1973 [1963]), p. 17.

[26] ibid., p. 15.

[27] Thurmann, *Samling af Love, Forordninger, kongelige Rescripter og Resolutioner, Placater, Reglementer, Instruxer, Fundatser og andre offentlige Aktstykker vedkommende Læger, Apothekere, Dyrlæger og Gjordemødre i Kongeriget Norge*, p. 34.

[28] See for instance Letter to Collegium Medicum from Deegen 27.3 1773 and 18.8 1774, State Archive in Kristiansand, Lister and Mandal county (hereafter: SAK).

[29] Adeler in a letter to Collegium Medicum 28.4 1774, RA (As in footnote 1).

[30] As a matter of fact this was not the first hospital for radesyge. An earlier hospital had opened in the main city of the diocese, Kristiansand, in 1763, but had to close in 1765.

[31] Rescripts of 3.6.1773, 21.12 1775 and 24.8 1774. In: L Thurmann, *Samling af Love, Forordninger, kongelige Rescripter og Resolutioner, Placater, Reglementer, Instruxer, Fundatser og andre offentlige Aktstykker vedkommende Læger, Apothekere, Dyrlæger og Gjordemødre i Kongeriget Norge*, pp. 34, 39 and 42.

[32] Moseng, *Ansvaret for undersåttenes helse 1603-1850*.

[33] On this aspect, see for instance Barbara Maria Stafford, *Body criticism : imaging the unseen in Enlightenment art and medicine* (Cambridge, Mass.: MIT Press, 1991).

[34] Laurence Brockliss og Colin Jones, *The medical world of early modern France* (Oxford: Clarendon Press, 1997), p. 672.

[35] ibid.

[36] Signild Vallgårda, *Sjukhus och fattigpolitik : et bidrag til de danska sjukhusens historia 1750-1880, Publikation / Institut for Social Medicin, Københavns Universitet 17* (København: Fadl, 1985), p. 18.

[37] Frederik Ludvig Bang, *Selecta diarii nosocomii regii Friedericiani Hafniensis* (Hafniae: Literis Simmelkiaerianis, 1789).

[38] *Interims Instruction For de til Cuuren af RadeSygdommen i Norge bestemte Candidater.* '[..]NB! Naar Candidaterne have havt et tilstrækkelig Antal af Syge under hænder, maa de samtlig indgive til Colleg. Medic. En omstændelig Efterrettning ikke allene om Sygdommens Beskaffenhed i sine adskillige grader men endog om de adskillige Cuur Arts Fordeel, Nytte, eller Inconvenience, samt om alt hvad der kand henføre til Oplysning om Sygdommens Aarsag, om Midler til at standse og udrydde den, og derefter skal den fra collegio blive tilstillet en nøiagtigere Instrux, og forholdes Ordre' 16.6 1774. RA (as in note 1)

[39] For instance in letter to Henrik Steffens 18.7 1775: 'dass Sie statt der letzten eingegebene Liste, über diejenigen mit der Radesyge behaftete Persohnen [...] eine Andere einsenden soll, wobey die Symptomata und Grad der Krankheit eines jeden Patienten, so wohl wie auch die verschiedene Cuur Arthen und deren mehr oder weniger glücklichen Ausfall angezeiget seyn sollen' RA (see note 1).

[40] See for instance Deegen in letter 5.10 1778, RA (see note 1)

[41] Steffens 22.7 1775 in report to Collegium Medicum, patient nr 9, RA (as in note 1)

[42] 'man udendes altid har anseet Hospitalers Oprettelse for det sikreste Middel til denne farlige Sygdoms ordentlige og fuldkomne Cuur, efterdi den Maade at curere den adspredt og hiemme i deres egne Huuse er langsom og utilstrekkelig, og derhos underkastet Vanskeligheter og Hindringer' Collegium Medicum to Amtmann Holm 15.8.1775. RA.

[43] See several letters from Collegium Medicum to the hospital doctors, e.g. 27.12.1776 to Henrik Steffens. RA.

[44] 'den täglichen gebrauche der Decoctum Mundificantium /:welche aus dem rad:Gramin:Taraxaci, Lign. Guajaci et Strobicul:pini bestehen:/' (Steffens to Collegium Medicum 29.6 1776).

[45] Steffens 29.6 1776. NA Pk 165 A-C.

[46] As for instance „Extr Trifol. Cochlear. Et Chinæ so in einem destil: afugelöset werden' Steffens 15.7 1775 NA Pk 165 A-C.

[47] Se for instance Deegen, letter to the King, 27.6 1777. SAK (as in note 26), Lister and Mandal Amts archive.

[48] Erwin Heinz Ackerknecht, *Therapeutics from the primitives to the 20th century (with an appendix: History of dietetics)* (New York: Hafner Press, 1973).

[49] See e.g. Claudia Stein, *Die Behandlung der Franzosenkrankheit in der frühen Neuzeit am Beispiel Augsburgs* (Stuttgart: Franz Steiner Verlag, 2003).. The leprosy hospitals in Norway also tried out medication on the patients from time to time in the 17th century.

[50] See Kari Blom et al., *'De fattige Christi lemmer': Stiftelsen St. Jørgens historie* (Bergen: Stiftelsen St. Jørgen, 1991). and Randi Kristin Strand, *Organisering av omsorg for spedalske under eneveldet: Reknes hospital 1708-1794* (Trondheim: Universitetet i Trondheim, 1997).

[51] Rescript to the county general in the County of Bratsberg, 24.8 1774, RA (jfr note 11) See also Pro Memoria by Hans Møller 4.8 1774. 'i Bratsberg Amt yttrer sig alt mere og mere den paa adskillige Steder i Norge grasserende saa kaldte Rade-Sygdom', RA (as in note 1).

[52] 'det vil være fornødent, for at see de med denne sygdom beladte mennesker helbredet, og forekomme sammes videre udbredelse, at et sygehuus der i amtet bliver foranstaltet opbygget' (ibid).

[53] 'sundeste og beqvemmeste Sted'. Rescript to the county governor in Bratsberg, Friderick Adeler, 24.8 1774,RA.

[54] 'til Doctorens Tieneste' (ibid)

[55] 'At befordre Sygehuusets Renlighed bade inden og uden Dørrs' (ibid)

[56] 'Lagnernes med de Syges nødvendige Tvæt og Vaskning, efter Doctorens Tilsyn og Begiering' (ibid)

[57] 'Ret efter Doctorens Instrux og overenstemmende med hans Cuurer'(ibid)

[58] 'maa og bestandig have tilsyn med de Syge, at de ey faar noget, som ikke af mig er bleven tilladt'. Henrik Steffens 20.8 1773 RA (as in note 1).

[59] See for instance Erik Pontoppidan: *Det første Forsøg paa Norges naturlige Historie: forestillende dette Kongeriges Luft, Grund, Fielde.* Kiøbenhavn 1752.

[60] Rachel Laudan, 'Birth of the Modern Diet,' *Scientific American* 238 (2000): 62-67.

[61] The National Archive, see several letters to the hospital doctors, for instance 27th of dec 1776 to Steffens op cit.

[62] Cited after Michel Foucault in Foucault, 'The Politics of Health in the Eighteenth Century', here p. 180. See also Foucault et al: *Les Machines à guérir: Aux origins de l'hôpital moderne.* Paris 1979.

[63] Michel Foucault: *The birth of the clinic.* London 1991, and William Bynum and Roy Porter: *Medical Fringe and Medical Orthodoxy 1750-1850.* London 1987.

[64] Moseng, *Ansvaret for undersåttenes helse 1603-1850.* Oslo 2003, p. 270

[65] See for instance Carl Wilhelm Boeck, *Traité de la Radesyge (Syphilis Tertiaire)* (Christiania: Johan Dahl, 1860).

[66] Ludwik Fleck, Robert K. Merton og Thaddeus J. Trenn, *Genesis and development of a scientific fact* (Chicago: University of Chicago Press, 1979).

Bibliography

Ackerknecht, Erwin Heinz. *Therapeutics from the primitives to the 20th century (with an appendix: History of dietetics).* New York: Hafner Press, 1973.

Arrizabalaga, Jon. 'Syphilis.' I: Kenneth F Kiple (red.), *The Cambridge World History of Human Disease*, s. 1025-32. Cambridge: Cambridge University Press, 1993.

Bang, Frederik Ludvig. *Selecta diarii nosocomii regii Friedericiani Hafniensis.* Hafniae: Literis Simmelkiaerianis, 1789.

Blom, Kari, Kjell Irgens, Egil Ertresvaag og Svein Aage Knudsen. *'De fattige Christi lemmer': Stiftelsen St. Jørgens historie.* Bergen: Stiftelsen St. Jørgen, 1991.

Boeck, Carl Wilhelm. *Traité de la Radesyge (Syphilis Tertiaire)*. Christiania: Johan Dahl, 1860.

Borge, C.J. 'Radesygen.' *Tidsskrift for den norske lægeforening* 25, no. 12 og 13 (1905): 427-32, 67-75.

Brockliss, Laurence og Colin Jones. *The medical world of early modern France*. Oxford: Clarendon Press, 1997.

Deegen, Henrik. *Noget om Radesygen, observeret ved Sygehuuset i Flechefiord og udgivet til Nytte for Almuen*. Christiansand: Andreas Swane, 1788.

Fleck, Ludwik, Robert K. Merton og Thaddeus J. Trenn. *Genesis and development of a scientific fact*. Chicago: University of Chicago Press, 1979.

Foucault, Michel. *The Birth of the Clinic: An Archaeology of Medical Perception*. London: Tavistock, 1973 [1963].

———. 'The Politics of Health in the Eighteenth Century.' I: Colin Gordon (red.), *Power/Knowledge: Selected Interviews and Other Writings 1972-1977 By Michel Foucault*, s. 166-82. New York: Pantheon Books, 1980.

Frank, Johann Peter. *System einer vollständigen medicinischen Polizey*. 2 utg. Mannheim: Schwan, 1784.

Frankenau, Rasmus. *Det offentlige Sundhedspolitie under en oplyst Regiering: især med Hensyn paa de danske Stater og deres Hovedstad: en Haandbog for Øvrigheder og Borgere*. København: Poulsen, 1801.

Hensler, Philipp Gabriel. *Ueber Kranken-Anstalten*. Hamburg, 1785.

Holst, Frederik. 'Sygehuse for venerisk Syge, Radesyge og andre ondartede Hudsygdomme i Norge i Decenniet fra 1822 til 1831.' *Eyr* 10 (1834): 1-44.

Hünefeld, Friedrich Ludwig. *Die Radesyge, oder Das skandinavische Syphiloid: aus skandinavischen Quellen dargestellt*. Leipzig: L. Voss, 1828.

Krünitz, Johann Georg. *Oeconomische Encyklopädie, oder allgemeines System der Staats-Stadt- Haus- und Landwirthschaft in alphabetischer Ordnung*. 242 bind. Berlin: Pauli, 1773-1858.

Laudan, Rachel. 'Birth of the Modern Diet.' *Scientific American* 238 (2000): 62-67.

Lie, Anne Kveim. 'Tanker om radesyken i Norge - 'den hentærer sine Offere langsomt'.' *Tidsskrift for den norske lægeforening* 123, no. 24 (2003): 3562-4.

Lie, Anne Kveim 'Radesykens tilblivelse.' Phd. thesis, University of Oslo, 2008.

Mangor, Christian Elovius. *Underretning om Radesygens Kiendetegn, Aarsager og Helbredelse*. Kiøbenhavn: Johan Frederik Schultz, 1793.

Moseng, Ole Georg. *Ansvaret for undersåttenes helse 1603-1850*. Bind 1 i Aina Schiøtz (red.), *Det offentlige helsevesen i Norge 1603-2003*. Oslo: Universitetsforlaget, 2003.

Reichborn-Kjennerud, I., I. Kobro og Fredrik Grøn. *Medisinens historie i Norge*. Oslo: Kildeforlaget, 1985.

Stafford, Barbara Maria. *Body criticism : imaging the unseen in Enlightenment art and medicine*. Cambridge, Mass.: MIT Press, 1991.

Statistisk sentralbyrå. *Historisk statistikk 1968, Norges offisielle statistikk*. Oslo: Statistisk sentralbyrå, 1969.

Stein, Claudia. *Die Behandlung der Franzosenkrankheit in der frühen Neuzeit am Beispiel Augsburgs*. Stuttgart: Franz Steiner Verlag, 2003.

Strand, Randi Kristin. *Organisering av omsorg for spedalske under eneveldet: Reknes hospital 1708-1794*. Trondheim: Universitetet i Trondheim, 1997.

Thurmann, L. *Samling af Love, Forordninger, kongelige Rescripter og Resolutioner, Placater, Reglementer, Instruxer, Fundatser og andre offentlige Aktstykker vedkommende Læger, Apothekere, Dyrlæger og Gjordemødre i Kongeriget Norge*. Christiania, 1851.

Utheim, John. *Oversigt over det norske civile Lægevæsens historiske Udvikling og nuværende Ordning, Bilag 2 til den kongelige Lægekommissions Indstilling*. Oslo: Johannes Bjørnstads Bogtrykkeri, 1901.

Vallgårda, Signild. *Sjukhus och fattigpolitik : et bidrag til de danska sjukhusens historia 1750-1880, Publikation / Institut for Social Medicin, Københavns Universitet 17*. København: Fadl, 1985.

Metaphors, Figures and Description in Sénac's *Traité de la structure du cœur, de son action et de ses maladies* (1749)

Eric Hamraouï

Abstract

In the two majors works *L'Anatomie d'Heister* (*Heister's Anatomy*, 1724 and 1735) and the *Traité de la structure du cœur, de son action et de ses maladies* (*Treatise of the structure of the heart, its action and its disease*, 1749), Jean-Bertrand Sénac (1693-1770) theorizes the interest of the correspondances, relays or shiftings of points of view settling more or less systematically between the text and the representation to make possible the multiplication of complementary information and the formulation of new questions. He allows an equal importance to the manifestation of the meaning by means of discourse and representation. In the two treatises, the use of metaphors also makes possible the semantic enrichment and the poetic pluralisation of our ways of feeling. However Sénac does not avoid the question of the veracity of the anatomical knowledge, owing to the 'endless turns' that our senses are compelled to follow to enable our mind to understand the 'mechanism' and the inner architecture of the human body.

Key Words: anatomy; figure; history of cardiology; metaphors; Sénac

*****

> *Il faut connoître la force et la puissance qui animent le cœur si nous voulons savoir comment nous vivons.*[1]
>
> We must first know the force and power that animate the heart if we want to learn how we live.
>
> Sénac

In his famous *Traité de la structure du cœur, de son action et de ses maladies* (*Treatise of the structure of the heart, its action and its disease*), Jean-Bertrand Sénac (1693-1770), the future first physician of king Louis XV, allows an equal importance to the manifestation of the meaning by means of discourse and representation. 'The expression of the image is just as decisive as the expression of the language',[2] he says. So doing, he contradicts the thesis of the native inferiority of the image, pale reflection or imperfect *mimesis* of the reality it pictures, compared with the text.[3] He also shows the impossibility to dissociate the analysis of the discursive forms (description, explanation), with the rhetorical figures (metaphors) combining with them to strengthen their persuasive power, from the study of the meaning provided by the anatomical representation with the gaps it sets in relation with the discourse that introduces, accompanies (legend) or comments it. But then, how can one define the modes of articulation of the two major forms of mediations between knowledge and practice that are *language* and *image* in Senac's treatise? A question in which the taking into account of this problem will lead us to endeavour to determine the manner in which the working in duality of text and image prevents the complexity of the reality that is scanned from becoming a source of confusion for the mind (the *vision* becoming *intuition*, the means of all knowledge and all thinking)[4] in absence of a technical instrumentation permitting to remedy the insufficient acuteness of our senses.[5]

1. Metaphors of the Life of Human Body

Sticking only to its medical aspect, with very few exceptions, historians of medicine have neglected the exploration of the philosophical and literary dimensions of Sénac's treatise. Concerning the philosophical point of view, I will not dwell on the materialist and at the same time vitalistic inspirations of the philosophy which is expressed in Sénac's treatise.[6] On a literary level, Sénac's book could be read as poetic praise of the heart, 'the material soul of the living bodies', similar to the praise of the wonders of creation contained in Johann-Jakob Scheuchzer's (1672-1733) *Sacred Physics or Natural History* (Zurich, 1733). Nevertheless, Sénac points out that the power of the heart also constitutes its vulnerability. He writes:

> *Mais le cœur est une espèce de centre où se réunissent tous les mouvements déréglés; tous les maux du reste du corps rejaillissent sur cet organe; dès qu'une partie est irritée ou enflammée, il en partage les souffrances; en les annonçant par un surcroît d'action, il y ajoute un surcroît de douleur, il porte le feu et le désordre partout.*[7]
>
> However, the heart is a kind of centre where all the irregular movements meet. All the ailments of the rest of the body flash back on this organ. As soon as any part is irritated or inflamed, the heart shares its afflictions. Announcing them by increased action, the heart intensifies them with increased pain; it carries the fire and the disorder everywhere.

The metaphors expressing both the centripetal and centrifugal diffusion of disease that affects the heart cited above, which Flaubert might have had in mind when he wrote that 'all the miseries of humanity can gather there [in the heart] and dwell there as its guests',[8] show that, in its description of the heart's deterioration, Sénac's treatise does not stop at the correlation between a perceptual sector and a semantic element.[9] The inventive richness of the description of elements of the structure of the heart by Sénac bear witness to this. He compares for instance the Eustachian valve to a 'kind of sling', or to a 'brake':

> [*une espèce de fronde ou un] frein qui attache la veine cave au trou ovale, la retient quand elle se remplit ou se dilate, la tire en se contractant [...], forme par sa partie large, un éperon, ou une digue plus ou moins grande, convexe quand elle est poussée par le sang, plate quand elle est affaissée.*[10]
>
> [a kind of sling, or a brake] that attaches the *vena cava* to the oval orifice, retains it when it fills up or dilates, pulls it while contracting [...], and forms a ridge, or a relatively large dam with its wide part, which is convex when it is pushed by blood, and becomes flat as it collapses.

Is it, as Aristotle thought,[11] because the word meant to signify the things – or the parts of the living body – in act can only do it by depicting them, that Senac has here recourse to the metaphor? Or are we to see in this recourse the consequence of the possession of a science allowing to recognize the similar in the dissimilar?[12] That science, which is at the origin of the creation of new relations of similarities, makes possible in its turn the semantic enrichment and the poetic pluralisation of our ways of feeling, as it is shown, according to us, in the description achieved by Senac of the agents and principle of the life of the human body: the nerves and the connection of the vital powers. 'Reins of the soul',[13] in the way that they give orders to the body, and 'primary springs of the animal machine',[14] the nerves contain the heart's animating principle in their invisible canals.[15] Although they are a prolongation and a continuation of the brain, they are not its instrument. Indeed, they posses their own principle of action.[16] Thus, they are similar to 'true brains', the seats of the formation, of the stationing, of the flow and action of the animal spirit:[17] hence their function as centres that distribute life in all the parts of the body. In short, the nerves are defined by Sénac as a 'vital source' whose flows meet those of the spinal marrow and of the cerebral substance. Moreover, for a time, they are able to compensate for the failures of the latter.[18]

According to Sénac, the principle of life consists in combined action, or 'circle of causes'[19] understood as 'the connection of the vital powers'[20] of the neural spirit, the heart's impulse, and the action of the vessels. The second vital power (the impulse of the heart) is carried to all the parts of the body by the arteries which Sénac defines as 'an extension of the heart'[21] and thus, as the 'real hearts distributed to each part and to each fiber.'[22] The latter metaphor holds the idea of a 'decentralisation' of the principle of life destined to become one of the key concepts of the vitalistic thought of the end of the 18th century.[23] So, far from betraying any weakening of reason, a distraction through images,[24] the activity of metaphorical re-description within the scientific discourse works fundamentally as imagination generator of concepts.[25]

2. Observing and Describing Diseases

Sénac's opens its words to the richness of perception. Hence the importance Sénac lends to the evocation of colour and texture of the organic alterations. He writes:

> *La substance des polypes ressemble au tissu d'une toile. Ce ne sont pas seulement les parties blanchâtres du sang qui se disposent en réseau, on trouve le même arrangement dans les parties rouges [...].*[26]
>
> The matter that makes up the polyps resembles the texture of linen. It is not just the white blood elements that arrange themselves in a network, we find the same arrangement in the red elements [...].

A few pages later Sénac compares the structure of the polyps to that of onions since they are both formed 'by an arrangement of various layers, one on top of the other'.[27] He also speaks of 'polyp beds'[28] in order to describe the clusters of blood or lymph that form in aneurisms. Indeed, he claims to have observed 'polyps with branches, or floating polyps'.[29]

Two sets of metaphors make possible the adaptation of medical language's logic to the nature of the alterations observed in the fourth book of Sénac's treatise, which studies the diseases of the heart.[30] The first set refers to the dynamic of the pathologic processes (metaphors of ignition, ordering and of motion the second set refers to the damages incurred by those processes (metaphors of exhaustion, of collapsing, of extinction and of overturn).

The metaphor of ignition describes the action of acute diseases that affect the internal parts of the heart,[31] as well as the inflammation of its internal walls.[32] The metaphor of ordering describes the continual, autonomous, and involuntary action of the nerves and of the heart or 'vital principle' that animates all of the springs of the 'animal machine'.[33] Sénac describes this animation as 'the motion of the animal spirit' driving the 'motion of the heart':[34]

> *La force qui agit alternativement dans les fibres du cœur [...] est une force qui s'éteint et qui renaît à chaque instant; elle produit à chaque seconde, ou plus souvent une secousse momentanée; le relâchement succède à chaque secousse, et une secousse suit chaque relâchement; cette succession de repos et de mouvement est la marche de l'esprit animal, ou de la cause mouvante qui est dans les nerfs ou dans les fibres du cœur.*[35]
>
> The force that periodically acts in the fibers of the heart [...] is a force that dies and comes to life again at each moment. Every second or more often, it produces a momentary jolt; each jolt is followed by rest, and one jolt follows each rest. This succession of rest and movement constitutes the motion of the animal spirit, or the moving cause that is in the nerves or in the heart's fibers.

The metaphors expressing the damage caused by pathological disorders are those of the exhaustion of the blood,[36] as opposed to its impetuosity [37] of the collapse of the pulse in certain fevers, of the ambivalence of the agents of life 'where nature sowed the secret causes for our destruction',[38] and finally, of the overturn (in the most catastrophic sense of the word) of the order of the body's functions in the case of neural damage.[39] The metaphor of extinction works to depict the fatal outcome of the, so-called, 'simple' diseases that attack one part of the body in particular.[40] This extinction of the vital spirit is not always irreversible, as is shown by the example of people that are brought back to life after drowning. Sénac writes: 'The principle of life survives [...] long after the appearance of death; it can thus reanimate the body when death seemed to have extinguished all the organ's work'.[41]

The metaphors Sénac uses sometimes contribute to the dramatization of the physiological or clinical observations reported. He writes for example:

> *Voilà, ce qui arrive au cœur lorsqu'il pousse un sang qui lui résiste ; cette résistance est comme un aiguillon qui agit sur les ventricules, & qui y cause un surcroît d'action.*[42]
>
> What happens when the heart pushes blood that resists it is that the resistance is like an arrow spurring the ventricles & producing an increase of action in them.

Sénac's clinical observations and reports sometimes take the same form as the 'narrative accounts' that focus on the more fantastic aspects of the disease. Thus, in the following passage, Sénac's language invokes the case of Saint Philip of Neri (1515-1595), who founded the Oratorians' Congrégation of Rome in 1564. Suffering from an aneurism of the heart and of the pulmonary artery, Saint Philip often felt violent palpitations following his states of mystical ecstasy:

> *Saint Philip de Néri étoit sujet à des palpitations si violentes qu'elles avoient détaché deux côtes de leurs cartilages; ces côtes s'abaissaient & s'élevoient alternativement suivant les divers mouvements du cœur; ce viscère avoit un volume extraordinaire ; le calibre de l'artère pulmonaire était double de celui qu'elle avoit naturellement.*[43]
>
> Saint Philip of Néri was prone to palpitations so violent that they detached two sides of their cartilage; these sides rise and fall alternatively, following the movement of the heart. This organ was extraordinarily large; the diameter of the pulmonary artery was double its natural size.

Similarly, Sénac recalls 'the case of an auricle as large as an infant's head on a person that surrendered to the fits of anger.'[44] Moreover, he describes the case of a heart 'as large as the heart of a bull', whose right ventricular valves contained 'a rock or tartary concretion the size of a chestnut'.[45] This last text implements a vivid combination of new relations of resemblance that contribute to semantic enrichment[46] – a poetics of the medical discourse on disease. However, the colorful portrait, and the description of the alterations and structure of the heart by means of analogy and metaphor which I have just cited as examples, do not yet bear out the displacement of the diagnostics toward the realm of an esthetic sensualism (Cabanis).[47] The sensualist method that uses all the senses to show that which, although given to perception, remains invisible or imperceptible, had not yet made its way into the field of medicine. Thus, in spite of the research diagnosing disease in the living patient (*intra vitam*) established by Lancisi (1654-1720), autopsy remained the single guarantor of the veracity for the diagnosis of diseases.

3. An Epistemological Ideal

In the two majors works that are *L'Anatomie d'Heister* (1724 and 1735) and the *Traité de la structure du cœur* – whose contents and images shall be resumed in the article 'Heart' of the *Encyclopedia* – Sénac theorizes the interest of the correspondances, relays or shiftings of points of view settling more or less systematically between the text and the representation to make possible the multiplication of complementary information and the formulation of new questions.[48] That wealth of information thus available grants to Sénac, according to the author of the recension of the second work, appeared in the *Journal des sçavans,* 'the glory of having revealed a real secret, a part of the structure of the human heart, that many an author have missed, and other have preferred not to undertake'.[49]

However Sénac does not avoid the question of the veracity of the anatomical knowledge, owing to the 'endless turns', that our senses are compelled to follow to enable our mind to understand the 'mechanism' and the inner architecture of the human body:[50]

> *La connoissance des parties du corps & les lumières de la Physique ne sont très souvent qu'une foible ressource: le volume, la figure, la situation sont presque les seuls objets qui se présentent à nos yeux; quand nous voulons suivre la nature dans le tissu des parties, nous foisons, il est vrai, quelques pas dans les grandes routes; c'est-à-dire que nous suivons le cours des gros vaisseaux; mais leur nombre ne reconnoît point de bornes, ils se dérobent bientôt à nos sens, & ils se plongent, pour ainsi dire, dans l'infini; c'est pourtant dans cet infini qu'il faut découvrir leur structure; si une industrie éclairée force quelquefois la nature à se découvrir un peu, elle nous présente de nouvelles difficultés dans ce qu'elle nous découvre; une structure grossière qui est le seul objet que nous puissions saisir en suppose toujours d'autres que nous pouvons seulement deviner; la*

> *ressemblance même nous en impose souvent, & c'est une source seconde d'illusions.* [51]

> The knowledge of the parts of the body & the lights of Physics are very often only a feeble resource: the volume, the image, the situation are almost the only objects that appear before our sight; when we want to follow nature in the tissue of the parts, we take it is true, a few steps in the main routes; that is to say we follow the course of the big vessels; but their number is endless, soon they are hidden to our senses, and they sink, so to speak, into the infinite; yet it is in this infinite that their structure must be disclosed; if a lucid ingeniousity sometimes compel nature to unveil itself a little, it sets in front of us new difficulties in what it discloses ; a gross structure that is the only object we can apprehend always leads us to suppose the existence of others within it, that we can only guess at; the very similitude often deludes us, and it is a second source of illusions.

In these conditions, how can one describe and represent the 'maze'[52] and 'the circle without any beginning or end' that appears to the eyes of whoever wants to study the structure and action of the parts of the human body? How can one cross 'the almost insuperable barriers' [53] that nature, only disclosing itself through its 'outside aspects' [54] or 'effects' [55] has set between itself and the observer? In fact Sénac writes:

> *La machine animale est comme le cercle qui n'a ni commencement ni fin; un ressort prête son action à l'autre qui lui doit son mouvement ; leur union conspire à former d'autres machines qui deviennent leur mobile ; enfin, tous les ressorts réunissent leurs mouvemens dans chaque ressort, & chaque ressort partage aux autres son action & ses productions.* [56]

> The animal machine is like the circle which has neither beginning nor end; a spring lends its action to another that owes it its movement; their union conspires to form other machines which become their mobile; in the end, all the springs gather their movements in each spring, and each spring shares with the others its action and its productions.

Are not these obstacles likely to entail in the anatomist an insurmontable distorsion between the act of *seeing* and the fact of *representing*? In order to prevent the latter risk, Sénac advises the respect of both these methodological principles. The first principle consists in the previous decomposition of the observation in several distinct stages:

> *Il est impossible d'[...] exposer [les nerfs intercostaux] aux yeux si on veut les disséquer ensemble ; ce n'est qu'après les avoir vus dans une longue suite de cadavres qu'on peut se former une image de toutes les distributions des divers entrelacements.*[57]
>
> It is impossible to [...] expose [the intercostals nerves] to the sight if one wants to dissect them together; it is only after seeing them in a long succession of corpses, that one can conceive an image of all the repartitions of the diverse intertwinings.

The second principle is this: the re-centring of the execution of each image on the representation of a particular aspect of the 'natural situation' of the heart or of its parts, in order to prevent any risk of confusion generated by the desire to make the representation more accurate than the anatomist really can.[58]

As nature alone detains the truth of our knowledge,[59] it is on the other hand necessary for the anatomist whose mind has a thousand motives to fall a prey to confusion and the senses as many motives to be subjected to illusion, to operate a de-multiplication of the points of view of observation.

> *Telle est la fécondité de la nature; elle présente toujours des objets qu'on ne cherche point et des replis qu'on n'a pas vus [...]; l'esprit est toujours surchargé de la multiplicité des objets, ils s'y déguisent même en s'y gravant; la mémoire ne rend qu'avec infidélité ce qu'on lui confie ; de même que les peintres tracent leurs portraits en suivant des yeux les traits qu'ils copient, j'ai décrit sur le cadavre même ce que je voyais ; mais les yeux ne sont pas moins sujets à l'illusion que l'esprit ; pour n'être pas séduit par l'imagination, j'en ai toujours appelé aux yeux des autres.*[60]
>
> Such is the fertility of nature; it always discloses objects that one does not look for, and folds that one has not seen

> [...]; the mind is always overloaded with the multiplicity of objects which disguise themselves even as they get engraved therein; memory gives back only unfaithfully what is entrusted to it; just as painters draw their portraits following with their eyes the features they copy, I have described on the very corpse what I saw; but the eyes are not less prone to illusion than the mind; to avoid being deluded by imagination, I have always appealed to the others' eyes.

But the complete objectivation of the anatomist's sight might not be obtained without having recourse to the reduction of the complexity of the object under observation, which Sénac here interprets pedagogically the result of by means of images and comparisons themselves anticipating on the contents of the representation that is figured:

> *Ce n'est que par la simplicité qu'on peut pénétrer dans ce qui est composé ; or pour simplifier cet assemblage de fibres si nombreuses et si diversement dirigées, il faut les réduire à trois espèces principales ; tout ce qui résultera de ces fibres pourra être appliqué aux autres.*
>
> *Soit donc un cône environné d'une fibre qui marche spiralement ; soit roulée autour d'elle une autre fibre spirale qui marche dans un sens opposé ; soit enfin entre ces deux fibres, une troisième fibre circulaire ; que doit-il arriver, si ces trois espèces de fibres viennent à se raccourcir?* [63]
>
> It is only through simplicity that one can penetrate whatever is complex; now to simplify this medley of fibres so numerous and so diversely oriented, one must reduce them to three main categories; all that shall result from those fibres can apply to the others.
>
> Suppose then a cone surrounded by a spiralling fibre; suppose, coiled about it, another spiral fibre that works in an opposite direction; and between those two fibres, a third circular fibre; what is to occur if those three sorts of fibres happen to get shorter?

The endeavour to increase the objectivity of the anatomist's look will in the end show, in a no less obvious manner, by attributing to the legend of the anatomical plate the role of critical instrument of the observation and of means of possible rectification of the mistakes of interpretation of the image.[61] The information contained in the legend has, according to Sénac, a value as a synthesis of the contents of the *description* based on the observation of the structure of the parts of the human body and of the *explanation* of the physical spring of their movement, founded this time on reasoning. The latter operation alone protects anatomy from the risk of being reduced to the status of topography of the areas of the human body, unable to represent the routes that run through them or allow one to have access to them: 'The knowledge of the structure of the parts without the lights of Physics is just a guide which only shows the names of the places one must travel through.'[62]

Clarity of the description and of the image, accordance (convergence) between the information revealed in both of them, coincidence between the accuracy of the former and the sharpness of the latter, such are, according to Sénac, the conditions of a rigorous knowledge of the anatomy of the human body. The formulation of the latter demands itself presupposes the recognition of a character no less meaningful to the representation than to the description of the parts of the human body.[63] Indeed, the 'ideas' of the anatomist suggested by the outline of the picture that is drawn, sometimes happen to be no less demonstratively expressed than in the discourse.[64] Thus Sénac mentions the ability of some anatomists to convey their ideas as if they had written them. About that, he quotes the example of Eustache's anatomical plates (1510-1574), which, long devoid of explanatory comments, were nevertheless 'monuments in which [that Anatomist had] engraved his ideas.'

Let's remark, in the end, that the images contained in Sénac's treatise don't serve only as *reference* to the text, but as *model* that the commentary must imitate:

> *Les descriptions doivent être comme les figures; tout l'objet qu'elles représentent doit y être tracé: si on omet une partie, quelque petite qu'elle soit, une proportion, ou une position qui paraîtra indifférente, on omet peut-être un instrument essentiel, ou une condition nécessaire: les plus petites parties entrent dans la composition du corps qu'elles composent, ou concourent à son action.*[65]
>
> The descriptions must be like the pictures; the whole object they represent must be drawn in them; if one leaves out a

> part, however small it be, a proportion or a position that may seem insignificant, one perhaps omits an essential instrument, or a necessary condition; the smallest parts enter into the composition of the body they compose, or concur to its action.

Avoiding the inconvenience of the words that have more 'outline' or 'boundaries' [66] than thought, and may be the support of the simultaneous expression of several ideas, the anatomical representation here is supposed to replace the description thanks to its ability to satisfy the double demand of exhaustion and the taking into account of the position of each element in space. Those demands aver themselves in conformity with the epistemological ideal of completeness of the elements of knowledge defined in the article 'Observation' of *the Encyclopedia*, published only a few years later.

4. Philosophical Stakes

The study of the nature of the relations between *discourse* and *representation* in Sénac's treatise has first enabled us to enhance the possible blurring of the frontiers existing between each of the two terms of the relation, by means of overthrowing the hierarchy usually ruling the relations of text and representation: the latter becoming the *model* of the former. The play of interactions and reciprocal transformations working between the material of 'descriptive figuration' [67] and the textual support, as well as the attribution of an archetypal function to the representation, produce of an 'accurate sensitive imagination',[68] thus form the two modalities of the didactic imposition of a perception, and the suggestion of a sense[69] in Sénac's treatise. In both cases is stressed an identical pursuit of accuracy and strictness, the repetition of the same processes of observation on different subjects, as well as the sense of detail, not for its own sake, but for what it reveals that was concealed, or for the links it enables us to establish with other details.[70] That exigency of accuracy at work as well in the theory of experience as in the theory of representation[71] leads us to come back briefly on the question of the foundation of the heuristic value of anatomical representation. The latter, doing violence to the native reluctance of things to be worded and to appear in the open,[72] introduces a qualitative differentiation between the *thing* as seen (the anatomy of the parts of the human body) and the *object* as represented (the picture).[73] So it can be defined as the instrument of en endeavour to unveil 'the carnal being of the depths' (Merleau-Ponty[74]), and to apprehend the unity of the living system 'that can be viewed and dislocated from the outside, but that can be understood only if one looks back to its hidden roots, and if one systematically follows the life whose impulse moves within them and springs from them, the life that gives the shape from the inside.'[75]

Translated from French to English
by Victor Hugo Velazquez
and Yolande Ricommard

Notes

[1] Sénac, *Traité de la structure du cœur, de son action et de ses maladies, par M. Sénac, Médecin consultant du Roy*, 2 vol. in-4°, Briasson, Paris, 1749, pp. 504, 694. 17 plates engraved on copper, drawn by Pottier, captain of infantry and engineer of Maréchal de Saxe, preface.

[2] ibid., I, p. 351.

[3] R Rey, 'Le cœur en représentation. Étude des rapports entre texte et représentation dans quelques ouvrages scientifiques du XVIIIe siècle' in *Interfaces,* Paris 1994, p. 181.

[4] Here we refer precisely to Kant's definition of intuition, on which begins the 1st paragraph of transcendental Aesthetics of the *Critic of Pure Reason*, 1781 and 1787.

[5] E Hamraoui, *Philosophie du progrès en cardiologie,* Éditions Louis Pariente, Paris 2002, p. 288.

[6] Sénac defines the agent of the body's movement as material principle and supposes the existence of one vital principle.

[7] Sénac, *Traité de la structure du cœur*, preface.

[8] G Flaubert, *Novembre*, presented and annoted by A Abensour, Librairie Générale Française (Le Livre de poche), Paris, 1840-1842, p. 42.

[9] M Foucault, *Naissance de la clinique*, P.U.F./ Quadrige, Paris, (1963), 1988, p. 173.

[10] Sénac, *Traité de la structure du cœur*, I, p. 431.

[11] Aristotle, *Rhetoric,* III, 11, 1411 b 24-25, crit. ed. A.Wartelle, Les Belles Lettres, Paris 1973: 'I declare that the words depict when they mean the things in act.'

[12] Aristotle, *Poetic*, chap. 22-59 a 6-8, ed J.Hardy, Les Belles Lettres, Paris 1932: 'The major thing is by far, the use of the metaphor ; that is the one thing that cannot be taught ; it's the gift of genius ; for by the right use of the metaphor, one is to see the similar.'

[13] Sénac, *Traité de la structure du cœur*, preface.

[14] ibid.

[15] ibid., I, p. 331 and 426.

[16] Sénac, *Traité de la structure du cœur, de son action et de ses maladies, par M. Sénac, Conseiller d'État, Premier médecin du Roi*, 2 vol., in-4°, 532 et 611 p., edition reviewed and et published by Portal, Méquignon, Paris, 1783, II, p. 516.

[17] ibid., II, p. 119.

[18] ibid.

[19] Sénac, *Traité de la structure du cœur* (1749), II, p. 262.

[20] Sénac, *Traité des maladies du cœur*, Bardou, Paris, 1778, p. 260.

[21] Sénac, *Traité de la structure du cœur*, 1749 and 1783, preface.

[22] Sénac, *Traité des maladies du cœur*, op. cit., p. 280.

[23] 'The vital principle is (...) the immediate cause of action in all the parts; therefore it is essential to each part and appears as the property of each one', thus speaks the surgeon John Hunter (1728-1793) in his *Lessons on the principles of surgery* (1774-1785). Also see O Keel, 'Les conditions de la décomposition analytique de l'organisme: Haller, Hunter, Bichat', *Les études philosophiques*, January-March 1982, p. 50.

[24] P Ricœur, *La métaphore vive*, Seuil, Paris, 1975.

[25] ibid.

[26] Sénac, *Traité de la structure du cœur*, II, 1749, p. 448.

[27] ibid., p. 451.

[28] ibid., p. 452.

[29] ibid.

[30] E Hamraoui, 'Visualisation et interprétation clinique des sons perçus par auscultation médiate chez R.T.H. Laennec' in *Philosophie*, n° 40, Minuit, Paris, 1993, p. 24-49.

[31] Sénac, *Traité de la structure du cœur*, II, 1749, p. 270.

[32] ibid., p. 381.

[33] ibid., p. 532.

[34] ibid., p. 325.

[35] Sénac, *Traité de la structure du cœur*, II, 1783, p. 23.

[36] ibid., p. 349.

[37] ibid., p. 383.

[38] Sénac, *Traité de la structure du cœur* (1749), II, 442.

[39] ibid., p. 309.

[40] ibid., p. 306

[41] ibid., p. 315.

[42] ibid., p. 269.

[43] ibid., p. 409.

[44] ibid., p. 401.

[45] ibid., p. 428.

[46] P Ricœur, *La métaphore vive*, Seuil, Paris, 1975, p. 240-41.

[47] O Keel, *Cabanis et la généalogie épistémologique de la médecine clinique*, PhD, Department of Philosophy, Mc Gill University, Montréal, 1977, p. 655.

[48] R Rey, *op. cit.*, p. 195.

[49] *Le Journal des sçavans*, Paris, January 1750, p. 478.

[50] Sénac, *L'Anatomie d'Heister avec des essais de physique sur l'usage des parties du corps humain*, Paris, J Vincent, 1724, 1 vol., pièces limin., 724 p.; 1735, p. viij-ix.

[51] Sénac, *L'Anatomie d'Heister* (1735), p. xiij.

[52] Sénac, *Traité de la structure du cœur, preface*, 1749 p. xj.

[53] ibid., p. xliv.

[54] ibid., I, p. 149.

[55] ibid., p. 289.

[56] Sénac, *L'Anatomie de Heister* (1735), p. ix ; *Traité de la structure du cœur* (1749), preface, p. xx ; I, p. 74.

[57] Sénac, *Traité de la structure du cœur* (1749), I, p. 119.

[58] ibid., p. 165.

[59] ibid., p. 10: Even though it is 'in its outside aspects like an obscure book that lends itself to all interpretations […]. Nature alone can show us truth'.

[60] ibid., preface, p. xviii.

[61] R Rey, *op. cit.,* p. 199.

[62] Sénac, *L'Anatomie d'Heister* (1735), p. viij.

[63] Sénac, Traité de la structure du cœur (1749), I, p. 351.

[64] ibid.

[65] ibid., preface, p.xii.

[66] V Hugo, *L'homme qui rit*, Ed. de la 'Librairie illustrée', Paris 1874.

[67] E Cassirer, Individu und Kosmos in der Philosophie der Renaissance, Teubner, Leipzig, 1927.

[68] ibid., p. 208.

[69] R Rey, op.cit., p. 181.

[70] R Rey, op. cit., p. 198.

[71] E Cassirer, op. cit., p. 208.

[72] F Dastur, 'À la naissance des choses: le dessin', proceedings of the Colloque de l'École des Beaux-Arts de Toulouse: 'L'art au regard de la phénoménologie', 25-26-27 May 1993, Presses Universitaires du Mirail, Toulouse, p. 90.

[73] Endowed with a 'phenomenological' sight, the draftsman is not content with passively registering of the thing. Leaving aside his ordinary vision, he makes it stand and spring as it is facing it, and constitutes it in an *object* outside consciousness (Dastur, op. cit., p. 76-77). Therefore appears the

character essentially inchoative of the fifured representation (ibid., p. 88-89).

[74] M Merleau-Ponty, *Le visible et l'invisible*, Paris, Tel Gallimard, (1964) 1986, p. 179.

[75] E Husserl, *La crise des sciences européennes et la phénoménologie transcendentale*, translated and prefaced by Gérard Granel, Gallimard, Paris, (1938), 1990, p. 129.

Bibliography

Aristotle, *Rhetoric*. Crit. ed. A.Wartelle, Les Belles Lettres, Paris 1973.

Aristotle, *Poetic*. Ed J. Hardy, Les Belles Lettres, Paris 1932.

Cassirer, E., *Individu und Kosmos in der Philosophie der Renaissance*. Teubner, Leipzig, 1927.

Dastur, F., 'À la naissance des choses: le dessin', proceedings of the Colloque de l'École des Beaux-Arts de Toulouse: 'L'art au regard de la phénoménologie'. Presses Universitaires du Mirail, Toulouse 1993.

Flaubert, G., *Novembre*. Presented and annoted by A. Abensour, Librairie Générale Française (Le Livre de poche), Paris, 1840-1842.

Foucault, M., *Naissance de la clinique*. P.U.F./ Quadrige, Paris, (1963), 1988.

Hamraoui, E., *Philosophie du progrès en cardiologie*. Éditions Louis Pariente, Paris 2002.

Hamraoui, E., 'Visualisation et interprétation clinique des sons perçus par auscultation médiate chez R.T.H. Laennec'. *Philosophie*, n° 40, Minuit, Paris, 1993.

Hugo, V., *L'homme qui rit*, Ed. de la 'Librairie illustrée', Paris 1874.

Hunter, J., *Lessons on the principles of surgery*, 1774-1785.

Husserl, E., *La crise des sciences européennes et la phénoménologie transcendentale*. Translated and prefaced by G. Granel, Gallimard, Paris, (1938), 1990.

Kant, I., *Critic of Pure Reason*. 1781 and 1787.

Keel, O., 'Les conditions de la décomposition analytique de l'organisme: Haller, Hunter, Bichat'. *Les études philosophiques*, P.U.F., Paris, January-March 1982.

Keel, O., *Cabanis et la généalogie épistémologique de la médecine clinique*. McGill University, Montréal, 1977.

Merleau-Ponty, M., *Le visible et l'invisible*. Tel Gallimard, Paris, (1964) 1986.

Le Journal des sçavans, Paris, January 1750.

Rey, R., 'Le cœur en représentation. Étude des rapports entre texte et représentation dans quelques ouvrages scientifiques du XVIIIe siècle'. *Interfaces*, Paris 1994.

Ricœur, P., *La métaphore vive*, Seuil, Paris, 1975.

Sénac, M., *Traité de la structure du cœur, de son action et de ses maladies, par M. Sénac, Médecin consultant du Roy*. 2 vol. in-4°, Briasson, Paris, 1749.

Sénac, *Traité de la structure du cœur, de son action et de ses maladies, par M. Sénac, Conseiller d'État, Premier médecin du Roi*. 2 vol., in-4°, edition reviewed and published by Portal, Méquignon, Paris, 1783.

Sénac, *Traité des maladies du cœur*. Bardou, Paris, 1778, p. 260.

Sénac, *Traité de la structure du cœur*. 1749 and 1783.

Sénac, *L'Anatomie d'Heister avec des essais de physique sur l'usage des parties du corps humain*. J Vincent, Paris, 1724.

Who's Afraid of Amalie Skram? Hysteria and Rebellion in Amalie Skram's Novels of Mental Hospitals

Hilde Bondevik

Abstract
In this chapter I intend to shed light on hysteria as a cultural diagnosis by examining two novels from 1895 which are set in mental hospitals: *Professor Hieronimus* and *På St. Jørgen,* written by the Norwegian-Danish author Amalie Skram. The discussion employs an understanding of hysteria as a typical illness and diagnosis of the time and as a form of hysterization of female disorder and rebellion. Amalie Skram and her life experience constitute a framework for the article, also suggesting that Skram may be regarded as an important figure in intellectual history that embodies the spirit of her age and helps to draft a new and modern female typology.

Key Words: Amalie Skram; disorder; hysteria; modern female typology; mental hospitals; rebellion

*****

At the conclusion of her book, Amalie Skram's first biographer, Antonie Tiberg, labels Skram as the ''great 'disease phenomenon' of her time'' (Tiberg 1910: 266).[1] With this comment, Tiberg suggests that Amalie Skram's encounters with 19th century psychiatry reflect wider, cultural issues. Rather than a narrowly defined medical case, the circumstances surrounding Skram's publication of her novels of mental hospitals. represent a privileged gateway into the conflicts and upheavals of her age, which often positioned women and their situation at the centre. In this way, 'she incarnated the spirit of her age,' as Inger-Lise Hjorth-Vetlesen points out (Hjort-Vetlesen 1993-1998: 467).[2] Thus Skram can simultaneously be read as a traditional case study and a case of medical history.

Because Amalie Skram was subjected to oppressive diagnoses, she became well-acquainted with the psychiatric practices of her age. Although the term is seldom used explicitly by Skram herself to describe the characters in her novels, the concept of *hysteria* is nevertheless frequently applied to both Skram herself and her fiction.

Several critics have identified instances of hysteria in Skram's fiction. The newspaper commentary from 1895 by physician Edvard Laurits Ehlers ultimately diagnoses the character Else Kant in *Professor Hieronimus* as suffering from hysteria: 'Mrs. Kant listens only to and pursues her hatred of

Hieronimus, and all the while documents her inability to master her own emotional life and displays a temporarily intractable, troll-like, purely hysterical disposition'.[3] Some of Skram's contemporary critics even relied on biographical information in their attempt to diagnose her fiction as hysterical, thus blurring biographical, medical, and fictional discourses. Hinting at Skram's case against the Municipal Hospital in Copenhagen, on October 14th 1894 the newspaper *København*, for instance, cites Amalie Skram's own medical history: 'every time she worked on a new book, the author was in a state of high tension and nervousness, at times hysterical'.[4] The attempts at categorizing Skram's fiction as hysterical do not, however, end with the 19th century. In her analysis of *Professor Hieronimus,* Unni Langås also suggests that hysteria is the central theme of Skram's book, which she sees as constituting an exemplary illustration of the diagnosis.[5]

The attempts at diagnosing Amalie Skram have been many. If we are, however, to take the author seriously, then perhaps the opposite may be the case? In contrast to the objectifying interpretative practices of most critics who have been interested in Skram and hysteria, I suggest that it is she who makes the diagnosis – of her own age, of women's positions, of marriage and of bourgeois society. Skram's novels therefore represent a diagnostic examination of society and culture in general, but especially of the way women and their bodies are treated in the Victorian ideology which characterized Scandinavian bourgeois culture at the end of the nineteenth century.[6] Rather than functioning as a purely passive and objectifying term, I propose that Skram's fiction utilizes hysteria productively. As I interpret Skram's 'case,' hysteria is synonymous with *opposition, rebellion* or *provocation*, and although her female character is clearly subjected to these processes, her resistance to the medical and masculine interpretative paradigms of hysteria nevertheless reveals an increasingly vulnerable masculine domination.

In the following discussion, I examine how in Amalie Skram's two novels of mental hospitals *Professor Hieronimus* and *På St. Jørgen* such a rebellious form of hysteria represents a form of discursive transition that oscillates between objectifying diagnosis, Skram's subjective experience of extreme distress and her rebellious discourse. Her reaction and experience with the psychiatric institutions of the 19th century and their implied misogynist views are therefore transformed into prose and produces prose. As part of my argument, I will describe several contexts that might illuminate this wider cultural function of Skram's autobiographical fiction, and attempt to shed light on hysteria as it may be interpreted in her two novels from 1895 – the same year that Breuer and Freud published their well-known work *Studies on Hysteria.*

In my opinion, the representation of hysteria in literature supplements the medical discipline's understanding of the same diagnosis, and together literature and medicine can provide a more complete (albeit ambiguous) picture of the hysterical body and hysteria as a cultural diagnosis. A 'cultural diagnosis' will in this text be understood in its broader sense, neither as an illness or disease directly induced by culture, civilisation or lifestyle, nor as an illness related to certain ethnic groups. Rather a cultural diagnosis is characterised as an illness which has some sort of a 'career': it emerges in specific historical and cultural contexts and submerges in others. Its trajectory is characterized by a complex historical formation or genealogy: although it might have a long and ancient history, it nevertheless becomes manifest in a variety of different forms and through different bodily and mental symptoms. A cultural diagnosis will therefore reflect the history and culture of its age and often be exposed through other means than conventional medical discourse, for instance through literature. In this sense, a cultural diagnosis will undoubtedly say something about its present time.[7]

1. Hysteria's Golden Age and Skram's Reception

The period between 1870 and World War I is often referred to as the golden age of hysteria. The popularity of the diagnosis was partly a result of the neurologist Charcot's work at Salpêtrière Hospital in Paris in the final decades of the 1800s.[8] Hysteria also experienced a similar golden age in Norway. The relatively large number of scientific articles and debates published in medical journals, the significant number of diagnosed cases of hysteria (which included both women and men), and the many literary representations of hysteria by authors, such as Bjørnson, Ibsen and, of course Skram, all testify to the cultural proliferation and significance of this diagnosis in a Norwegian context.[9]

In *The History of Sexuality*, Michael Foucault refers to the second half of the 1800s as the time when the 'hysterization of the female body' occurred (Foucault 1995: 115-116). As I understand Foucault, hysterization functions consequently to discipline and pathologize women. As discipline, hysterization allows for a comprehensive pathologizing of women who 'deviate' from normative femininity. In this way, the pathological expressions which characterize hysteria - the more or less powerful physical symptoms - can be read as a rebellion against the disciplining of the body. Hysteria thus becomes something more than an ordinary female illness: instead it expresses an unbearable social or cultural condition. The hysterization of the female body is therefore involved in various relations of power both within smaller social units, such as the bourgeois home, in which women are assigned certain, unalterable roles and characterizations, but also in larger discursive formations, such as societal and institutional structures. In all these relations of power, a masculine, patriarchal dominance might pathologize and segment deviation from and rebellion against normative femininity through the diagnosis of hysteria. Within this dynamics it is the patriarchy, in this case represented by the male bourgeoisie of circa 1895, which has both the right and opportunity to define something as pathological. This power to define indicates in itself the constructed nature of the disease. Similar to Professor Hieronimus's defining power in Skram's novel of the same title, medical and scientific institutions and their authorities are also part of a machinery which defines and 'produces' hysteria, a dynamic which at the same time also produces or reproduces 'gender'. Our concepts of femininity are reproduced through specific diseases. Although some men also were diagnosed with hysteria in this period, this illness was undoubtedly most closely associated with women. Metaphorically speaking, hysteria is feminine and the feminine is hysterical. Hysteria has etymologically, culturally and metaphorically always been linked to the female body. In this sense, as Elisabeth Bronfen also has suggested, hysteria only exists as an effect of several discourses: Hysteria has '[...] no autonomous and original identity outside its discursive formations'.[10]

In reading Amalie Skram's novels of mental hospitals, several possible interpretations of her texts emerge. Some of these perspectives overlap, and some arise from the author's engagement with her own age. In Skram's own time, the critical approaches were dominated by readings in which her novels were viewed as a form of political documentary, or as important novels that referred directly to the prevailing psychiatric conflict in Denmark in the 1890s. After this follows a long period with strikingly little interest in the author and her work. Skram was considered as not belonging to the Norwegian literary canon, but was in this period rather regarded as a second-rate author who, at best, had contributed with some good, realistic descriptions of Norwegian society. Later in the 1970s, and primarily owing to the feminist movement, there is a renewed interest in Skram. This approach can be characterized as feminist in a political sense. Its primary focus was on undoing the literary canon's forgetting of Skram, and only secondarily to contribute with new analysis of the works themselves. Partly inspired by this project, a fourth approach emerges, in which Amalie Skram is investigated as a biographical project, and which emphasizes both Skram's use of her own life in her literary work as well as the influence of her literary work on her artistic life. Finally, yet another approach is exemplified by critics who focus on her 'style' in the broadest sense. While most literary critics identify Skram naturalistic writer, her work nevertheless contains strong symbolic elements. This fourth approach has therefore often questioned what type of 'naturalism' Skram subscribes to. Regardless of approach to the novels (and there are even more), it is interesting, as I see it, that hysteria as such becomes obvious if emphasis is placed on the literary works' contribution to the cultural conception of the nature of women and hysteria.

2. 'Amalie Kant' – Hysteria's Literary Figure

In her portrayal of Else Kant in *Professor Hieronimus* and *På St. Jørgen*, Skram builds on her own shocking experience with psychiatric institutions. Skram herself had been admitted to the Gaustad Mental Asylum in Kristiania in 1877. Seventeen years later, in February 1894, she was voluntarily admitted for observation at the Municipal Hospital in Copenhagen, and then later transferred against her will to St. Hans Hospital. These events provide a significant backdrop for understanding the novels *Professor Hieronimus* and *På St. Jørgen*'s critical perspective of 19th century psychiatry. These two novels then also made Amalie Skram a central figure in the controversy surrounding psychiatric care which took place in Copenhagen in February 1894. One of the other protagonists in this drama was the then chief physician of Copenhagen's Municipal Hospital, Knud Pontoppidan. *Professor Hieronimus* and *På St. Jørgen* were romans à clef or central novels that were easily seen through, and there was no doubt who Professor Hieronimus' real life model was.[11] In her two novels, Amalie Skram unmistakably confronts the chief physician, Knut Pontoppidan. Both Amalie Skram herself – and her character Else Kant – refused to assume the classic patient role and came into conflict with the chief physician. By refusing this role, she therefore questions and undermines his omniscience and authority to decide and define. Like the sarcastic remarks made by the nurses in *Professor Hieronimus*, it is as if Skram's novels also asks: 'One should always believe the doctors, isn't that right, Mrs. Kant?' Repeatly the undisputable authority of medicine is underlined in the two novels, and the power of the great professor is not to be discussed: 'Hieronimus's advice must be followed'.[12]

Considering the intense public reaction Skram's books helped trigger, connected as it was to three other cases from *Copenhagen's Municipal Hospital* which all illustrated a profession and a treatment in some sort of crisis, and the personal defeat suffered by Knud Pontoppidan who had to leave the hospital, the famous psychiatrist could naturally not have anything but a negative view of Amalie Skram. He responds to her fictional attack by exploiting his supposed 'impartiality.' When commenting on her novels, Pontoppidan states:

> It gives a realistic portrayal of how a mentally ill person's hateful indignation twists her mind and imparts to her distorted notions. She is not capable of giving an objective account.[13]

Perhaps ironically does Pontoppidan's accusation point precisiely to Skram's main discursive method? Skram's writing is in many ways characterized precisely by opposition, rebellion and provocation. This opposition, which manifests itself as a type of unrest, disorder, hysterical behaviour, and which in this sense can be understood as a type feminine writing, is countered by the physician's diagnosis. Interestingly, Skram portrays her opposition to the infantilization, divestment of self-determination, and objectification of woman - or simply, to the hysterization of herself, by exploiting the productive, discursive potential of hysteria .

When one of the best known Norwegian authors of the time, Bjørnstjerne Bjørnson, asks Skram to write about her experiences 'as they were,' and moreover, to explain the background in equally realistic terms, Skram's text approaches the genre of autobiography:

> You should unconditionally portray it exactly as it is. But you must also depict (or at least mention) the circumstances that led you there. Otherwise they will use it to harm you. You must show clearly what will be too much for you. Why you yourself asked to be placed under Pontoppidan's observation. Then you will have a foundation for the rest. Promise me this! And write like thusly![14]

Bjørnson writes this in answering Skram's letter of 22th April 1894, posted at the St. Joseph's Hospital in Copenhagen. Her letter represents more than a personal message to a dear friend, instead it constitutes the first draft of the novel about Else Kant. In Amalie Skram's letter to Bjørnson, she tells of her difficulties with writing, and how this leads her into a condition that she herself describes as a type of infirmity: 'I could not manage to write the book, (it is always *therefore* I become ill) [...]', something which adds to the many symptoms Skram herself displays: insomnia, coughing, lack of appetite, crying fits, which consequently supplement and confirm the notations in her medical journal.[15] From this point on, the journey to her admission to a mental hospital is short. In her letter, Skram complains about her problems and describes how she agrees to undergo treatment. It is here it all begins. Skram's letter to Bjørnson constitutes her first discursive experiment with these events. The following quotation from Amalie Skram's letter to Bjørnson represents in itself a summary of *Professor Hieronimus* and *På St. Jørgen*:

> Then I said to Skram: This will not work; let me take a short break from my work, because if I continue on like this, just staring and staring at it, I think I shall go mad in

> the end. Yes, I shall. Then S. met with our doctor and came to me and said: Have you any objection to being admitted to the Municipal Hospital under Pontoppidan for one and a half week's time to speak with him and listen to the advice he has to offer you? 'No,' I answered. 'Not in the slightest. To the contrary,' - and left calmly, but I should not have done so, for then I marched straight into hell. S. left me with the promise that he would return to see me every other day [...][16]

The statement that she would go 'mad' and march 'straight into hell' points to her experiences with the psychiatric institution, while the account of her husband's somewhat deceitful and less than chivalrous behaviour ties into the novel's plot. She emphatically rejects the notion that she is insane or in any way mentally ill, just as her character Else Kant does later in the novel. Skram begins that same letter to Bjørnson with these words: 'I have not been more insane now than you have been! But I have been confined and abused as if I were a dangerous lunatic [...].' The 'letter of farewell' that Amalie Skram writes to Pontoppidan concludes with these words: 'For all this and more, as soon as I am released from Blidstrup, the Professor shall be held accountable in a public forum. Quickly and at the last moment, your sincere enemy!'[17]

In this light, Skram's narrative reproduces reality. The disorder of hysteria stands in stark contrast to the order of medicine or psychiatry, and in all its formlessness refers to a production of something new. Here creation and production do not have identical meanings, understood as taking shape or gaining an identity, but rather signify something unpredictable, that something which does not yet exist or in this sense to discursive potentiality. In the conclusion of *På St. Jørgen,* Else Kant enters an uncertain future, which suggests that her process, both in medical and the discursive sense, is ongoing and open-ended. She is still on the verge of becoming what she will become. In other words, the novel projects the nature of hysteria as a type of productive disorder onto a future space where the novels about Else Kant may be read as a description of timeless, female self-realization.

The correspondence between Skram's letters and novels, understood as the stylistic and thematic exchange between the two genres, clearly points to an autobiographical affair. The parallels between Amalie Skram and Else Kant are more than obvious: they mirror each other. In other words: They are not the same, but a reflection of the same.[18] Elaine Showalter goes one step further in her interpretation of Skram when she writes in the introduction to *Under Observation* that Else Kant is a projection of Skram: 'She is clearly an autobiographical projection of her creator'.[19]

But the novels about Else Kant were nevertheless understood as true descriptions of conditions in the Danish psychiatric institutions, and aroused intense reactions. Her novels were considered by many readers to be 'authentic documents,' which of course they were not, if one by this understand her novels as neutral reports of the conditions in these psychiatric institutions. On the other hand, the novels are obviously 'authentic' and truthful in the sense that they are accounts of an experience. The dual status of Skram's mental asylum novels as both realistic literature and autobiographical fiction at the same time, underline therefore the complex relations between real-life experience and prose.

3. Hysteria as a Critique of Subjectivity

Clearly, neither *Professor Hieronimus* nor *På St. Jørgen* constitute autobiographies in the strict sense. But the issue is not so simple: the 'self-biographical' generates certain fundamental problems which are highly significant in this case. According to Philip Lejeune, who has written several books about autobiography[20], a kind of 'contract' between the author and the reader is needed in order for an autobiography to exist. A crucial component in this 'contract' is that the author 'signs' her name to the book's title. One of Lejeune's most important critics is Paul De Man, who writes that Lejeune's position is tied up in the notion of a *guarantee* and *confirmation* of the written subject.[21] In this lies a critique of the stability and permanence of subjectivity and of the assumed unambiguous and unique quality of identity, an approach which is associated with the almost canonized list of modern and post-modern critics. But without evoking the entire spectrum of a hermeneutic of suspicion from Marx, Nietzsche and Freud up to our time, I propose that in her two small novels about Else Kant, Amalie Skram writes autobiographical prose that can be read as a critique of subjectivity, in which hysteria functions as a significant tool. For it is precisely through the hysterization of the female, understood here as the diagnosis of Skram/Kant as mentally ill, insane, unsound, etc., that the notion of the unambiguous, permanent and, ultimately, 'masculine' identity expresses itself most powerfully. The critique of this aspect of hysterization is the most important element of Amalie Skram's asylum novels. Skram's productive, discursive use of hysteria to critique hysterization, echoes one of the most influential readings of *Professor Hieronimus* and *På St. Jørgen*, namely that in her novels of mental hospitals Skram finds a solution to her own artistic crisis.[22] In this way, Skram's experiments with discursive hysteria in *Professor Hieronimus* and *På St. Jørgen* represent an emerging modernism, not only because of her critique of the masculine, authoritarian discursivity and methodical subjection of women that take place in these psychiatric institutions, but also because of her critique of the notion of an unambiguous identity.

4. Hysteria's Dialectic Between Symptoms and Signs

In her two novels, Amalie Skram describes female, mental illness, but more importantly, how female patients interact with a patriarchal, authoritarian institution. The protagonist in both novels, the painter Else Kant, starts out in a comfortable bourgeois marriage, but after a period of exhaustion and little sleep, as well as after having experienced great frustration with her own work, she reluctantly agrees to submit to psychiatric observation. There she encounters an almost violent institution and a cruel physician, Professor Hieronimus. Striking at this point is that Else Kant, in her own eyes and as she is primarily - but not exclusively - described, seems healthier when she passes the threshold to the asylum, rather than before. In the opening of the novel, her illness seems to fit the diagnosis of hysteria as it was defined in much of the medical literature of the day. According to 19th century definitions of hysteria, some of the most important symptoms included an inexplicable cough, insomnia, dizziness, heaving convulsions, and nervous twitches, followed by an inability to move, stiffness, and fatigue. Skram's protagonist experiences many of these: 'Else lay motionless. Her head burned but otherwise her whole body felt dead, except when sudden, spasmodic twinges in her chest made her jump with pain'.[23] The above list of symptoms is, however, not complete. Medical literature frequently supplemented and expanded their definitions with yet new forms and expressions of hysterical conditions to make the diagnosis fit even more cases and symptoms. In this sense institutional treatment and observation can be said to provoke and produce new symptoms of hysteria. In Skram's novel, the main activity Else Kant engages in at the asylum, however, is a thorough and analytical observation of the institutional conditions. This 'project' draws her out of her suicidal thoughts and depression, and transforms her angst to indignation and anger. Suicide is not a suitable solution, not only because of her husband, Knut, and her son, Tage, but because she would not be able to testify about the shocking conditions at the institution: 'If she could escape alive, she could tell her story – warn, and perhaps save, even one fellow being from the things she had experienced. No, she *had* to live' she concludes.[24]

In light of this, it is also possible to read Else Kant's symptoms as part of a hysterical condition which is defined by a dialectic of opposition: she opposes a world which has put pressure on her, and she is subjected to further, institutional dominance. In a sense it is therefore precisely Else Kant's 'sanity,' which not unexpectedly causes her to rebel against the institution and the physician's authoritative figure which then the doctor interprets as signs of a difficult, obstinate patient, and ultimately a hysterical woman:

> – 'You are quite hysterical, you know.'
>
> – 'How could a person in here be anything else?' Else continued, twisting in agony. 'It is inexcusable, inexcusable'.[25]

Through Else's reply, Skram illustrates the constructed nature of hystery, or how the institution is involved in reproducing its eclectic symptoms. This is again suggested by how Kant, after her encounter with the physician, experiences even more symptoms of hysteria. Kant's inexplicable cough persists, she cannot move as she wants, and she is sometimes stricken by spontaneous muteness: '[…] her throat was so constricted she could not utter a sound'.[26] She is also afflicted with dental pain, which is clearly inexplicable, yet all the while she refuses to see a dentist. Else Kant also has hallucinations, and thus loses her composure now and then. She gives in somewhat, and calms down, but this is also typical of hysteria. Gradually, she acquires symptoms which clearly indicate that they are provoked or produced by the mental institution; this is especially the case when Else Kant is subjected to a form of treatment that was known as 'confinement.' This method involves mechanical means of stripping the patient of her right to self-determination and autonomy. Even Else's husband, Knut, questions (for once) this de-humanizing treatment. When Hieronimus decides that Else Kant will be transferred to St. Jørgen's Mental Hospital 'for a period of time – not too brief' – he estimates a one-year stay, Else's husband asks:

> – And it's your opinion that this will really produce a cure?
>
> – Without reservation. We have had many instances of it. The first six months will pass under protest from your wife. Then she will quit down, and eventually leave the hospital with gratitude in her heart, quite cured (ibid.: 87-88).

It is this confinement, or 'treatment,' that Skram describes as causing Else Kant's breakdown. But in spite of this: Else appears gradually as something else or more than broken, or rather, the breakdown itself has created something new: '[s]he felt battered and shaken, but at the same time, strengthened' (ibid.: 124). If one is satisfied with a list of symptoms as a diagnostic criteria of hysteria, Else may seem sicker than she really is, or more aptly put, her symptoms may overshadow the fact that her 'illness,' also is a product of and simultaneously a rebellion against a misogynistic institution. Else's insight into her own 'illness' is therefore significant, just as the solidarity among the women in the asylum also points beyond its walls. What Skram's novels illustrate is that hysteria can resist hysterization by communicating with the world outside, but that it does so in a language that expresses itself through signs of illness and a form of rebellion which others attempt to pathologize.

Unlike Else Kant's hysterical discourse, Hieronimus remains inside the asylum walls. He repeatedly suspects that Else Kant is lying about her afflictions. At one point he also suggests that her hysteria is more than a 'small' hysteria, and that she rather has displayed signs of the Charcotian *grand hysterie,* as exemplified when he says to her: '- You used to throw yourself naked on the floor, writhing and howling, isn't that correct?' (ibid.: 156). Else resists this suggestion by replying that she certainly has never been naked. According to Hieronimus' masculine reasoning, hysteria is part of an erotic imaginary, as it was in Charcot's definition of *grand hysterie.* In contrast to Charcot, the father of modern hysteria, Hieronimus understands hysteria as also including force and abuse, or a form of a sadistic Eros. Hinting at this particular form of sadism, Else puts him in the same category as 'the executioner who delights in his work' (ibid.: 156).

Another little discussed, but interesting aspect of the novels is Else's dreams, which technically operate somewhere between hallucinations and actual dreams. Sometimes in this dream-like state, a number of animal figures appear, such as horses, lions, tigers, dogs, and roosters. From a Freudian perspective they read as signifying repressed, yet overpowering sexuality. Her dream about the parade of the beautiful, brown, blind horses at the beginning of the novel has thus been interpreted as a sign of sexual angst (Lyhne), or as a picture of an artistic crisis (Engelstad) (Lyhne 1981: 76, Engelstad 1992: 203). It is, however, perhaps possible to also understand the dream of the galloping horses – supplemented by the conception of wild animals, lions, tiger, wolves and dogs – as figures associated with flight, or a form of identification (a *devenir-animal*)[27] that the imagination can use to sketch for itself a freer or different life form, a way of being pointing toward an emancipation from a human reality which has become too constricted - or human, all too human. This is also confirmed by how the institution 'sees' Else. The rebellious, wild nature that characterizes Else Kant's dreams and imagination fit well with the institution's reaction: '- Oh yes indeed, she was watched and peered at like a strange animal'.[28] Interpreted this way, Else is a woman with significant talent, with a visual power to represent, and an ability to rebel. In this way, her dreams also become part of a reality-producing, critical position. Hysteria's expressive mode rebels against a particular type of masculine domination that Skram's novels represent by the ways in which psychiatric institutions position themselves as having the distinctive authority to define 'human.'

5. Hysteria as Disorder's Rebellion against Masculine Domination

By using an ordinary, but sickly female protagonist and subjecting her to an uncomprehending, male-dominated institution, Skram evokes a critical potential. What she criticizes is both the psychiatric institution's treatment of patients as well as society's treatment of women, as represented by the institution of bourgeois marriage. Even though her husband, Knut, has some critical observations of the psychiatric system, he is totally supportive of putting Else's fate into its hands. The same is true of their family doctor, Tvede, who supports the Professor in everything, as well as the associate specialist, of course. In this way, Skram also criticizes another institutional hierarchy of power, namely, the relationship and struggle between the various medical positions, from the family doctor and associate specialist, up to the institution's chief physician and Professor. In addition, it is also symbolically interesting to note the solidarity among the women, such as when Else, for example, is escorted by women in and out of her next hospital stay. Her stay at St. Jørgen, however, becomes completely different than expected. The confinement she experiences here dissolves her from within. Yet this has a productive and revitalizing potential: broken, but strengthened, she walks out of the asylum restored to health.

Read with an eye for a new approach toward the author's aesthetic orientation toward a new and productive use of experience, hysteria in Skram's work does not just function as illness. Instead, the formlessness which characterizes hysteria may be read as an immanent part of subjectivity, because it illustrates how subjectivity is always in process, in a state of continual change and becoming. In this way, the twin novels *Professor Hieronimus* and *På St. Jørgen* may be read with an eye for *life*, not death, or in other words, with a focus on that which seems to be moving toward something new and better.[29] Else Kant, in this sense, is therefore not merely ill, just as Hieronimus should not only be read as dangerous, monstrous and evil. Within an interpretative framework which critique institutions, he appears as a natural villain, but because of his exaggerated monstrosity and lack of credibility, the Hieronimus figure appears instead as laughable and inflated to the point of the comical. Skram exposes the type of power and mechanisms that produce hysteria as an 'illness' through a rhetoric of exaggeration. In contrast to an attempt to eliminate or annihilate the power of hysterization only through direct criticism, Skram also makes it appear laughable.[30] This type of strategy to counteract power – the attempt to make superior force and abusive power appear comical, is accounted for with great clarity by Skram herself. In this way, Skram's depiction of institutional power is not only a question of tragedy, sacrifice and suffering, but it is also a manifestation of the crisis of power. Her critique of the degrading and inhuman conditions of these psychiatric institutions, also reflect an inner crisis of power which made these conditions possible in the first place.

Else Kant should not necessarily be regarded as ill, just as her sexuality should not necessarily be understood as repressed. Instead, Else's hysteria displays a fluid, suggestive sexual desire, a 'coming into existence,' which more than anything else functions as a *devenir-woman*, a process, or a path toward realization. The important intellectual historical figure that she in fact constitutes lies in the fact that she shows with great clarity how a new humanness takes shape, namely, as a new authority, a new self. While psychiatrist and Skram biographer Borghild Krane concludes that Skram does not 'predict a new and free female typology,' I would not agree with this conclusion, since Skram's prose is certainly more ambiguous and complex than readings à la Krane would indicate.[31] Hysteria raises objections and questions by being radically ambiguous, but then it is also radically unmanageable. It is here that the unmanageable nature of hysteria is accounted for - hysteria's disorder juxtaposed against medicine's order.

Owing to its inconsistent and disorderly nature, Skram's hysterical discourse can be read as a rebellion against masculine domination, rather than signifying unsatisfied female desire. Perhaps what Skram shows us is that hysteria represents a greater challenge than what modern diagnostic schemes would indicate? There are not just a few authorities with a distinctive 'power to define' that may feel threatened by a literary figure such as Else Kant or, for that matter, the now canonized author Amalie Skram.

Notes

[1] A Tiberg, *Amalie Skram som kunstner og menneske*, Aschehoug Forlag, Kristiania, 1910, p. 266.

[2] All the Danish and Norwegian quotations are translated by the author of the article.

[3] M Gradenwitz, *Knud Pontoppidan og patienterne: Etatsraaden, Sypigen, Amalie Skram, Grevinden*, Akademisk Forlag, København, 1985, p. 71.

[4] ibid., p. 62.

[5] U Langås, 'The Struggle for the Body – Hysteria and Rebellion in Amalie Skrams Novel *Professor Hieronimus*', in *Scandinavian Studies*, Nr. 1, vol. 75, Provo, UTAH, 2003, p. 58.

[6] In a Norwegian context some of the plays of Henrik Ibsen illustrate this sort of Victorian ideology and women's positions of bourgeois society – especially *A Dolls House* and *Hedda Gabler* which also could be read as plays that stage hysteria, see Hilde Bondevik 'Henrik Ibsen og hysteriet', *Edda* 4/05.

[7] See Johannisson, 1990 or Hacking, 1999.

[8] About 'hysteria's golden age' see e.g. Mark S. Micales *Approching Hysteria: Disease and Its Interpretations* (1995), which is one of the most well written, learned and comprehensive study of the history of hysteria and its historiography. See also Elaine Showalters classical book *The Female Malady: Women, Madness and English Culture, 1830-1980* (1987).

[9] See Hilde Bondevik, *Medisinens orden og hysteriets uorden. Hysteri I Norge 1870 – 1915,* phd-thesis Universitetet I Oslo, Unipub, Oslo, 2007.

[10] E Bronfen, *The Knotted Subject. Hysteria and Its Discontentes*, Princeton University Press, Princeton, 1998, p. 102.

[11] See Vagn Lyhne, *Eksperimentere som en gal. Psykiatriens sidste krise*, Modtryk, Århus, 1981, page 9. See also the book reviews and newspaper coverage in connection with the case, as accounted for in Mogens Gradenwitz (1985).

[12] Skram, 1992, p. 88.

[13] Gradenwitz 1985, p. 73.

[14] B Bjørnson og A Skram, (ved A Øyvind og B Edvard) *'Og nu vil jeg tale ut', 'Men nu vil jeg også tale ud': brevvekslingen mellom Bjørnstjerne Bjørnson og Amalie Skram 1878-1904*, Gyldendal, Oslo, c1982, letter 61.

[15] See, e.g., *'Og nu vil jeg tale ut',* letter 48. Here Skram writes of her nervous cough and opium drips.

[16] ibid., letter 48.

[17] Gradenwitz, 1985, p. 57.

[18] Antonie Tibert writes: 'The portrayal of state of Else Kant's soul is an accurate reflection of Amalie Skram's at that time.' According to Tiberg, Amalie Skram was overworked, tormented by many tasks, housekeeping, childrearing, troubles with maids, and in particular, her own aesthetic project.

[19] Skram, 1992, XII.

[20] P Lejeune, *Le pacte autobiographique* Seuil, Paris, 1975.

[21] P de Man, Autobiography as De-Facement, in *The Rhetoric of Romanticism*, University Press, Columbia New York, 1984, pp. 71-72.

[22] I Engelstad, *Sammenbrudd og gjennombrudd. Amalie Skrams romaner om ekteskap og sinnssykdom*, Pax Forlag A/S, Oslo, 1992, p. 176.

[23] Skram, 1992, p. 104.

[24] ibid., p. 103.

[25] ibid., p. 62,

[26] ibid., p. 77.

[27] For more on the concept of 'devenir-animal', see G Deleuze and F Guattari, *Mille plateaux*, Minuit, Paris, 1980, pp. 284-380.

[28] Skram, 1992, p. 183.

[29] Skram's language is surprisingly modern; short and concise. The novels *Professor Hieronimus* and *På St. Jørgen* are relatively short. But why *two* novels when just one would have sufficed and perhaps carried more weight? One about the evil institution, the other about the good hospital? Or is it the time pressure due to the tempo of the political debate that leads Amalie Skram to publish the books one after the other? Are there financial motives? Is the division into two separate works a picture of a general dislocation, in which names and persons are changed or manipulated? A split novel?

[30] This approach to Kafka, which has inspired me, may be found in Gilles Deleuze and Félix Guattari, *Kafka, pour une littérature* mineure, Minuit, Paris 1975; Norwegian translation: *Kafka, for en mindre litteratur*, Pax, Oslo 1994. See also the foreword to the Norwegian edition, by Knut Stene-Johansen.

[31] B Krane, *Amalie Skram og kvinnens problem*, Gyldendal, Oslo, 1951, p. 173.

Bibliography

Bondevik, H., Henrik Ibsen og hysteriet, *Edda* 4/05.

Bondevik, H., *Medisinens orden og hysteriets uorden. Hysteri I Norge 1870 – 1915,* phd-thesis Universitetet i Oslo, Unipub, Oslo 2007.

Bjørnson, B. and Skram, A., Anker Ø. and Beyer E. (eds), *'Og nu vil jeg tale ut', 'Men nu vil jeg også tale ud': brevvekslingen mellom Bjørnstjerne Bjørnson og Amalie Skram 1878-1904*. Gyldendal, Oslo, c1982.

Bronfen, E., *The Knotted Subject. Hysteria and Its Discontentes*, Princeton University Press, Princeton, 1998.

Deleuze, G. and F. Guattari, *Kafka, pour une littérature mineure*. Minuit, Paris, 1975, Norwegian translation: *Kafka, for en mindre litteratur*. Pax Forlag A/S, Oslo, 1994.

Deleuze, G. and F. Guattari, *Mille plateaux*. Minuit, Paris, 1980.

Engelstad, I., *Sammenbrudd og gjennombrudd. Amalie Skrams romaner om ekteskap og sinnssykdom*. Pax Forlag A/S, Oslo, 1992.

Foucault, M., *Seksualitetens historie I, Viljen til viten*. Exil, Gjøvik, 1995 [1976].

Gradenwitz, M., *Knud Pontoppidan og patienterne: Etatsraaden, Sypigen, Amalie Skram, Grevinden*. Akademisk Forlag, København, 1985.

Hacking, I., *The Social Construction of What?*. Harvard University Press, Harvard, (1999), 2001.

Hiorth-Vetlesen, I.L., 'Lidenskabelig naturalisme. Om Amalie Skram', i *Nordisk kvindelitteraturhistorie*, bd. 2, 'Faderhuset', Møller Jensen, E. (ed), Rosinante/Munksgaard, København, c1993-c1998.

Johannisson, K., *Medicinens øga. Sjukdom, medicin och samhälle – historiske erfarenheter*. Nordstedts Förlag, Stockholm, 1990.

Krane, B., *Amalie Skram og kvinnens problem*. Gyldendal, Oslo, 1951.

Langås, U., The Struggle for the Body – Hysteria and Rebellion in Amalie Skrams Novel *Professor Hieronimus*. *Scandinavian Studies*, Nr. 1, vol. 75, Provo, UTAH, 2003.

Langås, U., *Kroppens betydning i norsk litteratur. 1800-1900*. Fagbokforlaget, Bergen, 2004.

Lejeune, P., *Le pacte autobiographique*. Seuil, Paris, 1975.

Lyhne, V., *Eksperimentere som en gal. Psykiatriens sidste krise*. Modtryk, Århus, 1981.

Man, P. de, 'Autobiography as De-Facement'. *The Rhetoric of Romanticism*, University Press, Columbia New York, 1984.

Micale, M.S., *Approching Hysteria: Disease and Its Interpretations*. Princeton University Press, Princeton, 1996.

Pontoppidan, K., *6. Afdelings Jammersminde*. Th. Linds Eftf., København, 1897, printed also in Mogens Gradenwitz.

Showalter, E., *The Female Malady: Women, Madness and English Culture 1830-1980*. Virtago, London, 1987 [1985].

Skram, A., *Under Observation* [*Professor Hieronimus* and *På Sct. Jørgen* 1895], translated from the Norwegian by Katherin Hanson and Judith Messick. Introduction by Elaine Showalter, Women in Translation, Seattle, 1992.

Tiberg, A., *Amalie Skram som kunstner og menneske*. Aschehoug Forlag, Kristiania, 1910.

Like a High Black Wave
Jørgen Stein and the Spanish Flu

Mette Kia Krabbe Meyer

Abstract

In 1918 the world faced a challenge as the great influenza swept the shores and lands of all countries. Scientists struggled to define the disease and citizens experienced a change in interpersonal relationships due to the fear of infection while they at the same time lived through sicknesses and deaths of dear ones. The Danish writer Jacob Paludan includes the influenza in his novel *Jørgen Stein*, a novel which, when published in 1932, was heralded as a factual description of provincial Denmark at the time of World War I. As one reads the book today, however, it becomes clear that its realism is a sticky affair. As to the influenza, the doubts, the grief and ethical dilemmas of the epidemic do, to a large extent, give way to a definition of infection which runs along the lines of the moral and sexual taboos established in the description of syphilis in cultural and literary history, for instance in the works of Thomas Mann. Paludan thus offers an account which is more or less a story of dubious culprits and scenes of crime. If the novel is to be regarded as a factual description of the influenza and its psychological consequences, my argument will be that is just as much due to the fact that it manifests a certain cultural reaction to the influenza, as it gives a detailed description of the epidemic.

Key Words: Epidemics; literature and medicine; Spanish flu

*****

At the end of the First World War, Denmark and the rest of the world was hit by the influenza epidemic known as the Spanish Flu. The epidemic came in three waves during the summer and autumn of 1918 and the beginning of 1919. In Denmark, the National Board of Health estimated in 1920 that a total of 710.000 people had been hit, and 11.400 of them succombed to the illness, according to two epidemilogists in 1991. Despite the large proportion of survivors, the unknown disease was considered extraordinarily frightening.[1] Medical science's triumphs at the end of the 19th century – particularly bacteriologists' successful attacks against a number of infective illnesses – had raised hopes of effectively fighting diseases.[2] The epidemic's extensive rampage was a blow against those hopes. During the epidemic, one lived with suffering and loss, but also with the danger of infection and restrictions. The public health system was put to the test, both scientifically and institutionally. Doctors were willing to treat, but really did not know what to use against the disease.[3] The State on one hand wanted to prevent infection, but on the other did not want to spread panic or inhibit functioning of the economy. The public were afraid of the disease and needed explanations, but also had a strong sense of being under attack from nature, leading to conflicting feelings from fear of close contact and a need for isolation to desire for company and to take care of one's ill family and friends. The epidemic created a great deal of tension in relationships between the individual and society, the economy and the disease, the biological definition and the psychological experience.

Jacob Paludan's contemporary novel *Jørgen Stein* portrays the period around the First World War, and thus the time of the influenza's outbreak. When the second part of the work was published in 1932, critics were united in calling it a realistic description of society and mentality. Tom Kristensen observed that *Jørgen Stein* offered a picture of 'the spirit of homey Denmark from 1914 to 1933', indicating the high measure of authenticity in the depiction of the latest things in fashion and popular music.[4] Indeed, all that contemporaneity was almost too much, wrote Kristensen, as characterization came to suffer under it. Later commentators also noted that characteristic of the book. For example, Ernst Frandsen wrote that Paludan 'can lift whole bits of perceived reality out of the past', while Orla Lundco maintained: '*Jørgen Stein* is also our newer literature's most significant bildungsroman, and with its placement in time – emphasized both in the overall concept and in the details – it dares demand to be counted as its era's most valid depiction of the time and place. *Jørgen Stein* is simply *the* book about Danish life between the wars.'[5]

However, any reader expecting a painstaking description of the Spanish Flu ravaging the period on the basis of the critics' appraisals of the novel as a realistic depiction will be disappointed. The depiction of clothing styles, musical refrains and newspaper headlines does not include face masks, rules of conduct to prohibit infection or article titles such as 'Lung plague'. That is not to say that the influenza is completely missing from the novel. It is described, but in my opinion Paludan gives influenza classic disease constuction, wherein infection is linked to moral ruin and the alien. As in Thomas Mann, a demonic South is constructed, where diseases come from, and infection is described as partly morally and partly erotically conditioned,[6] for example by putting it together with syphilis, which, beyond tuberculosis, had a nearly hypnotic effect in the period, as Michel Vovelle points out.[7] The aim of this article is to characterize Paludan's cultural blame-laying, which also has a geographic and political nature, but also to provide insight into the irresolution that reigned during the epidemic, which can be seen as having provoked the need for geographical and moral bases as a reaction. There were other ways of conceiving and describing the flu, both during the epidemic and in the subsequent literature. Albert Camus, who had sketched a general epidemic experience in *La Peste*, provides an example of conserving and exploring the uncertainty and ethical dilemmas that are nearly absent from Paludan's bourgeois bildungsroman.[8]

1. The Right Stuff in a Clan

Generally speaking, sickness and death in *Jørgen Stein* are woven together in a theme of ruin that owes a lot to Thomas Mann's philosophy of decadence.[9] One can draw a parallel between the Buddenbrook and Stein clans as strong family dynasties, both threatened by an unavoidable economic, spiritual and physical weakening, but whereas the Buddenbrooks go under, the Steins just do save their skin. At the start of the novel, we hear of the 'strong red Stein life blood' and of a family of the right stuff.[10] The good health is associated with the various personages' appearance and facial traits. It is emphasized, for example, that district revenue officer Hertz, who belongs to the Steins' circle, has a 'sharply chiseled English aristocratic' head.[11] Erik, who is lodged in the same place as Jørgen in Ålborg, is described on the contrary as a big, awkward, sluggish-looking fellow, which must correspond to his intellectual capacity.[12] Of course, Plaudan often puts the physiognomic interpretation into the mouths of characters, as in the case of Hertz, who closely follows Jørgen's development.

> District revenue officer Hertz was a thoughtful man, interested in faces and fates, and while he studied Jørgen, who had always seemed rather introverted, he asked himself how much of a share of the Steins' power that pale last-born had indeed inherited. No lineage's reserves were inexhaustable. …In decline they carry a sure sign that there was the right stuff in a clan.[13]

On the strength of Hertz's thought comes a suspenseful and angst-filled expectation of the Stein's decline, which great work of destruction begins with the outbreak of the war, as suggested by the title *Thunder in the South*.

The pale last-born, Jørgen, leaves his parents and comes, as mentioned, to Ålborg, where he and Erik are lodged in the home of piano dealer Aagesen. Here he becomes attached to the daughter of the house, Nanna, who like him is taken to have bad health, and they develop an affectionate relationship, but the attraction cannot measure up to the magnetic power over Jørgen of such dangerous women as the coffee seller's daughter, Ellen, and others. In a moment of destiny later in the novel, when Nanna has come to Copenhagen to visit him, Jørgen makes a decisive misstep. He cannot tear himself away from Ellen, and Nanna waits in vain for him and ends up going to a pub with a stranger. It is on that occasion that she is smitten with the Spanish Flu, and one can say that the flu, as it appears from the following, is also 'smitten' by Paludan's novel construction.

2. The Spread of Influenza

One first hears of the Spanish Flu when the young writer Femmer and Jørgen are taken to a market town inn, where they sit discussing literature, world politics and love. Femmer advises Jørgen to choose the healthy Nanna, whom he has just abandoned, and the two young men decide to go to Nanna's in order to provide Jørgen 'a human anchoring'. Paludan describes how the two grope their way out to get breakfast and a car and are met by a little woman who shushes them. The innkeeper is sick and the woman says, 'Shh. Shh. He's dying. There's Spanish Flu here'.[14] The influenza is thus depicted as something foreign that could concern Jørgen because he needs to see the innkeeper, and not because it could be a threat within his family. No letters have come from Havnstrup with bad news, and Jørgen's brother Otto – who like the former has also moved to Copenhagen by that time – is also fit and healthy. In is curious that the influenza's spread is just being realized. The formulation 'There's Spanish Flu here', says that the disease is not something one 'catches'. It is obviously not a disease one lives with and has as a part of one's personality, either. It is a disease that **is**, that strikes many and in some cases kills. Already in the first passage a self-contradiction is suggested in the novel. On the one hand the disease is described as a phenomenon of broad impact, but on the other hand there seem to be very few cases, in this place the innkeeper's and later the foreign travelling salesman's and Nanna's.

The contradiction is realized later in this passage from later in the novel:

> Like a high, black wave the Spanish Flu had suddenly risen up and rushed from the south toward Denmark; panic gripped everyone in those days. Whether its coincidence with war and fatigue was a matter of chance, no one knew, but it was like a tribulation, sent to teach both the healthy and the neutral fear, to teach them that no one should consider himself safe.[15]

The description could be extended to apply more generally to a view of the pandemic in the West as a critique of civilization. The circle is widened via channels in the infrastructure of modernity, for as Michel Foucault and Paul Virilio point out, modern life is characterized by higher and higher levels of intimity and speed.[16] In 1918 there was a constant circulation of money, goods, information and people in a great communications structure via the post, railroads, ship traffic, etc., and since the pandemic spread most easily where there were many people, it amounted to an attack on modernity. From a progressive, optimistic point of view, infrastructure and entertainment were considered positive, but the influenza turned mobility and intimacy into something demonic. In Crosby's dramatic formulation, 'We were all, so to speak, sitting in the waiting room of an enormous clinic, elbow to elbow with the sick of the world'.[17] One can find occasional examples of such a threat being mentioned in the Danish general public. A letter-writer to *BT,* signing as 'The still unsmitten', describes the Central Station as Dante's Inferno, for example. The station is tight-packed with people on no real errands, klumped together in groups, playing the accordian and singing loudly. When a stream of travelers approaches, according to the letter-writer, 'a metre-thick fog sits over the entire hall', and the air is 'foul-smelling and stifling'.[18] In the rationed society, where staple goods were scarce, one could read the following in the 'Snap-shot' of the day: 'That's what Hansen says, otherwise nothing is imported here; but cholera, that we can have as much of as we like. Same for the Spanish.'[19]

In the fall of 1918, when Nanna presumably presents the illness, influenza patients were constantly taking up more space. At Bispebjerg Hospital, the illness penetrated the 'healthy sections' in the baths building, the massage hall and machine shop, and so they had to refuse patients who were lying deathly ill in their own homes. Newspaper headlines read: 'The epidemic is now visible in the city', 'The Spanish Flu continues to spread' and finally 'All things considered, there will soon be hardly a work place, a business, a home where the 'Spanish Flu' has not gained entry [; W]ith this appearance it has erupted much more intrusively into social relations than it did last summer'.[20] The House of Parliament was even taken over as a hospital, and bodily metaphors for the whole city's condition were common currency. In *Nationaltidende*, for example, one could read, 'While the city lies comatose'.[21] The hospitals were as congested as flu victims' lungs, while other 'organs' lay empty. In Copenhagen many newspapers gave impressionistic portraits of rmpty palm courts, variety shows and restaurants, nor did Ålborg 'look so much like itself',[22] as Paludan writes of the city when Jørgen, in the fall of 1918, returns to visit the ill Nanna. As she lies sick under the second wave in autumn, there are ambulance alarms in the streets, the hotel he lives in is perhaps closed, the same for the variety show he reads about in a local paper, full of accounts of the epidemic. It is remembered by many Ålborgers, for example Egon Vandrup Jensen, who writes in his memoirs that 'Many young people could not make it through the disease; there were often whole pages of obituaries in the newspaper'.[23] Seen from a topographical viewpoint, one could note a radical change in the urban image, that naturally changed living conditions fundamentally, but it is a change that Paludan circumvents in his description of the influenza. The use of the wave as a metaphor really does not shift attention from the individual, guilty disease carrier and the epidemic that strikes humanity as an autonomous instance. The influenza's ravages are described only in Nanna's body, and therefore it is not really seen as a divine judgement, with reference to another description Paludan gives of the disease in the short passage. Such judgement does not function as an explantion of the disease's widespread damages, as it does in the contemporary *Kristeligt Dagblad,* for example.

3. The Disease's Breeding Ground

The wave metaphor was borrowed from the war, where it referred to the column or ring of smoke that spread out after a bomb explosion, and the metaphor could have caused Paludan to use influenza as an argument in defense of pacifism, as done by the left in Sweden.[24] In Denmark, the *Socialdemokraten* of 30 June 1918 noted that an influenza epidemic had broken out among German troops, and traced the disease's ravages among the soldiers in sick bay without taking the opportunity to criticize the war.[25] *Folkets Avis* was the quickest to mount a crusade against the church, upon which it pours sarcasm for remaining open while entertainment venues have been closed for fear of contagion.[26] That the contagion was connected to the war was correct, as contemporary research described how troop transporters functioned as disease transmission vehicles, while the war devastated national economies and limited the possibilities for antibiotic and contagion research.[27] Paludan might have made more of the connection between the war and the epidemic – given that the former is a central theme in the book because the generational conflict is expressed in disagreement between the nationalistic, militaristic County Commissioner and the young pacifist Jørgen – but it remains only a suggestion in the short interrogative passage.

The army is not made into a disease carrier, but is nonetheless a significant scapegoat figure in the novel. The wave comes from the south, and the notion of the South as the breeding ground of disease is naturally supported by Paludan's consistent use of the name 'Spanish Flu' instead of the neutral influenza. That the influenza came from the south was obviously correct in the case of Denmark, insofar as it was often spread via Germany. But that is part of the story – later clarified – that all European destinations were really just way stations, and the influenza can be traced to North

America.[28] That the disease came to be known as 'Spanish' is supposedly due to there having been no strong press censorship in Spain, as there was in the warring nations, France and Germany, and although the disease presumably came from America, the word of a mysterious disease came out of Spain. This means, of course, that the disease's name was locally given, and that the term became a normal name for the influenza can be taken as an indication of an ethnocentric folk culture. In Japan, for example, it was called the 'Flanders Flu'.

Generally the geographic designation serves to create a sense of security, a fixed point of reference, but obviously also a placing of responsibility. Instead of seeing the epidemic as a worldwide phenomenon, one focuses on its point of origin. The disease is referred back to a sort crime scene, and with it a number of perpetrators who can be blamed for it.[29] The phenomenon is old, since originally 'influenza' was a kind of astrological designation, placing the blame on other planets, inasmuch as Domenico and Pietro Buoninsegni, Italian historians who coined the word in 1580, were convinced that people's health was governed by the stars.[30] In the meantime, assigning responsibility has taken a less extraterrestrial turn. In the case of the Spanish Flu, there were, for example, rumours spread internationally that the epidemic was a part of German bacteriological warfare. However, Margareta Åman, who has thoroughly described the influenza's spread in Sweden, that scapegoats were sought to only a very limited extent.[31] One can certainly find caricatures, for example, the cartoon in *Ekstrabladet* from 23 October 1918, where some Spaniards are chasing Chief Medical Officer Axel Ulrik. But there are also many examples of pointing out the misleading nature of national designations, as in the *Socialdemokraten* article 'Influenza, the so-called Spanish Flu'[32].

Paludan, on the contrary, belongs to that faction that points to the South as the disease's breeding ground, which in the overall novelistic construction is linked to danger and ignorance. There is a suggestion of a social critique in the comparison to a divine judgment, doubt of any connection with the war and not least of all in the disease's connection with commerce and traffic. The critique is not, however, expressed in a broad description of the influenza's damage, and the various ethical dilemmas it poses for the population. This is due to the novel's form as a family chronicle rather than a large social portrait, and to the infection's status in the novel as a partly moral and sexual construction.

4. Infection and the Erotic

The linking of influenza and the erotic is a classic phenomenon. Not just sexually transmitted diseases, but a long list of ailments were seen as a result of sexual contact, including the Spanish Flu, which was also known as 'the Spanish Lady'. It is indeed curious that that name caught on at all, since it must have quickly become clear that the disease was not only caught from sexual contact, but from ordinary droplet infection. In that sense it is a good example of how some classic disease constructions with little to do with reality are activated. The name perhaps says most about the desire to find a causal connection and give the disease a body and gender.[33] As for the Danish press, there are not so many examples of a gendered, personified depiction. It was typically cartoonists who most frequently used personification. In a cartoon in *Politiken*, for example, the angel of peace is combined with the Spanish death in a kind of madonna–whore figure. The illustration had stuck in the memory of Dr. Harry Heidemann, who despite his familiarity with the disease's doubtful provenance and its wide geographic scope, reproduced the personification of the Spanish Flu in another drawing a year and a half later.[34] In Heidemann's version the Spanish Lady has become a skeletal figure – in *Politiken* she was a blend of skelton, tiger and woman. Heidemann also gave her a scythe over her shoulder, and he kept her provocative pose, not with a bare leg this time, but with a bare shoulder. She is flanked by two men, a syndicalist and a sailor, who represent the other threats to bourgeois order and family, namely the working class and sexually transmitted diseases.

In *Jørgen Stein* the threat to the Steins' health comes first and foremost from prostitutes, and throughout the novel father and son fear the venereal diseases flourishing in the city's underworld. The old county commissioner is afraid that his trembling hand is a symptom of syphilis, the result of a fateful bordello visit long past.[35] Young Jørgen visits a prostitute for the first time along with his friend Leif, but both father and son escape with only the fear. A Wassermann test exonerates the commissioner, to his and the family doctor's great relief, and Jørgen flees in terror from the prostitute Rita, with a scarlet-painted mouth, who would greatly like to take his innocence. Sexuality is thus linked to moral decay and punishment by sickness and death. Of course, Jørgen steers a somewhat unsteady course around the women who can lead him to ruin, both the prostitutes and summer acquaintance Lily, petite and fine featured, but with the same death's sign as the prostitutes – dark shadows under the eyes. Lily comes to the Steins' summer residence at the Vesterlyng Inn along with her father, a foreign professor who has made a discovery of 'dark nature' and has been married to a woman of 'foreign blood'. It is unknown whether she is Polish, Jewish or Estonian, writes Paludan. Tom Kristensen describes her as 'the colorful foreign butterfly…with Semitic shading on her wings', and there is no doubt that Lily is a Paludanesque version of Clawdia Chauchat, who in *Der Zauberberg* turns the head of young Castorp. In Mann's novel Chauchat has the role of the dæmoness, Lilith, found in Jewish folklore and *Faust*, and the allegory becomes even more evident in Paludan, thanks to the name Lily.[36]

It is neither Lily nor the prostitutes who bring the Spanish Flu into the Steins' circle, but sexual contact still plays a part. Nanna is no Zolaesque Nana, but she, too, undergoes a fall when, in a moment of weakness, she accompanies the stranger to the pub. The description of how she sought cover behind a plaster figure takes on a symbolic meaning when she discovers that it consists of a 'large, naked, rugged plaster leg' and comments that 'It was as if everything were bewitched' while the middle-aged stranger, like a Mannsk Aschenbach, makes careful, melancholic advances to her.[37] Thus, Nanna catches the influenza in a compromising situation as a result of Jørgen's indefensible treatment, since it was his absence that provoked her to go with the stranger. At the same time, it is her weak constitution that results in her becoming a fatality of the illness. Like Jørgen, who at the beginning of the novel must go to bed because he has got cold and wet feet on a walk in the woods, Nanna becomes ice cold in the rain while waiting for Jørgen, and her weakened body is the ideal growth medium for influenza. She must succumb because she has gone astray, but also because she does not have enough resistance and lets herself be led by her vision of death rather than fight the illness, as Jørgen urges her to do in the moment of truth. Whereas the linkage of infection and moral ruin is wrong, a strong immune system is an important weapon in the fight against the disease. It should be added, however, that a strong immune system in people who died of viral lung infection immediately after being infected was more an enemy than an ally. According to Collier and Barry the immune system went so hard on the attack against the virus in these cases that the war between the attacking cells and the virus turned the lungs into a dysfunctional battlefield.[38]

At the pub where Nanna is infected, the mystery deepens, since the infection is not just associated with moral deacy, but with destiny as well. Nanna faints when she recognizes the stranger from a vision has had in Jørgen's room. He has strawberry blond hair and dark shadows under his eyes, as do all the destructive figures in the novel. The result is that Nanna dies and her death comes to symbolize the death wishes of Jørgen and his clan. The wicked girls survive and the healthy girl perishes, and Jørgen continues to attract destruction until the end. The influenza has caused Nanna's slender round figure to dwindle, and Jørgen is taken with her meager, fragile body with the blue-grey shadows under the eyes that remind him of the 'loose women'.[39]

5. Insecurity and Fear

Aside from connecting the influenza to southern Europe and to the erotic, Paludan also depicts the Spanish Flu as a sure diagnosis. He makes the doctor an authority who calmly examines patients, and this give no impression of the irresolution that reigned among Danish doctors. As Lene Otto describes it, there was great frustration over the disease's mysterious ways, as concerned both diagnosis and treatment.[40] Bacteriology had given the medical profession firm ground to stand on, as they no longer just treated symptoms, but could also make microbiological diagnoses and treat patients with serums and therapy. Oluf Thomsen, Department Head at the National Serum Institute, identified typhus, Weil's disease, volhynia fever, infectious intestinal diseases, etc., but influenza could not be identified as a bacillus.[41] There was indeed a theory that the influenza was due to Pfeiffer's bacillus (*Haemophilus influenzœ*), but this was not accepted, and it was not until 1933 that the influenza became clinically defined.[42] Thus, during the epidemic many different symptoms were reported and there was great disagreement over whether the disease should be categorized as an influenza or not. Doctors grasped at all sorts of potions and expedients, from camphor to blood-letting in hopes of making a difference and halting the disease. It was a real crisis, where the only certain advice was that patients should take to their beds, and one might well wonder whether the doctors' constant running round among them did more to spread the disease than to tame it.[43] In Paludan's novel there is no description of the dead end doctors felt themselves trapped in. Contrary to nurses, who could follow their calling and care for the sick, doctors were unable to diagnose and cure, and that intolerable situation is the turning point of both Icelandic novelist Gunnar Gunnarson's *Salige er de enfoldige* (Blessed are the simple) and Albert Camus' *La peste*,[44] in both of which the doctors are challenged to define how to live with suffering as a basic condition, and fight – often in vain – agaist sickness and death.

While the hunt was on for the diseases cause among the microbes, various precautionary measures were also put in place. Few places implemented such strict quarantine policies as Samoa, where Commander John M. Poyer isolated the population from infections. Crosby[45] approvingly describes the authority Poyer wielded, and notes that democratic government can be a serious hindrance in an epidemic, when radical social inteventions are required. While this may be true, it is also clear that a strict quarantine program was a fata morgana when countries lay side-by-side like the world's organs, with traffic arteries running among them. Behavior modification thus became an alternative. Ortner Leichenstern had already written in 1905:

> He who is able to isolate himself from human intercourse, to prevent every contact with influenza patients, or with persons having to do with influenza patients, has to some

> extent a guarantee, similar to those inmates of certain prisons and strictly closed convents of escaping influenza.[46]

While Leichenstern counted on partial protection, the Dane Oluf Thomsen thought that behavior modification could act as kind of virtual quarantine. In *Berlingske Tidende* he describes how rather small, often invisible droplets can convey meningitis, polio, influenza, diptheria, scarlet fever, throat infection, tuberculosis, plague, etc., attacking those who are not vigilant.[47] The sick shoud cover their mouths when they cough, avoid singing or talking loudly, maintain a one meter distance from those to whom they speak, avoid touching objects others must touch and change handkerchieves frequently. Thomsen also says that exhalations themselves are not contagious and do not fill the room with bacteria-bearing droplets (the miasma theory), so one might go into sickrooms and aid the sick without danger. One should just avoid direct contact with infected droplets, and Thomsen concludes:

> Many will surely still find some of the mentioned measures exaggerated or laughable and yet the fact is that is everyone could and would observe them, the disease in question would disappear in one blow from the face of the earth, and we could concentrate on other enemies of life and health. Especially in public places, in trolleys and rail cars, in church, the theater and cafés people are incomprehensibly indifferent; they cough and sneeze into the air, and the mentioned places therefore become to the highest degree breeding grounds for the spread of infection during epidemics.[48]

This article and others from the period generally show that Danish doctors took the floor in the public debate, and there is thus no basis for the charge of silence that Wilfried Witte and Nancy K. Bristow level at the German and American medical professions, respectively. According to the authors, the lack of a medical explanation and cure meant that physicians and authorities avoided speaking about the illness. Witte writes:

> The Majority of the medical profession, together with the politicians and government public health officials, hoped that oral evidence would not survive for very long in a literate society and wrote about the influenza epidemic only when medicine and politics could not cope with the situation. A public discussion was not desired, the public was to be quiet.[49]

If it is misleading to represent medical science as a repressive institution, it is meanwhile appropriate to be critical of Thomsen's representation of the fight against disease. One could well ask if it were so simple vanquish the disease as he implies. The rabid proclamation testifies to Thomsen's powerful typical-for-the-era belief in improved hygiene as the answer to all of society's problems, but the article does not several problems into account. First of all, one could be a carrier of the disease without knowing it, so the rules of conduct applied across the board. Second, it was very difficult to avoid droplet infections. The face masks in use did not have the desired preventive effect, and this was linked to the risk of caring for the ill, leading to a fear of close contact that was caricatured in the contemporary press. The newspaper *København,* for example, let its two regular column figures, Fru Hansen and Fru Peddersen, go over the influenza in their chatter. In July they spoke most often of Fru Jensen, lying ill at home, and Ophelia may not look after her, as her husband is afraid of contagion. Neither may Fru Hansen go over there and get 'breathed on in the face'.[50] The popular understanding of cause and effect is also ridiculed when Hansen confides to Peddersen: 'But nowadays you have to be afraid, Fru Peddersen, that's one of the most important things! People who go around afraid and such, they have it easiest'.[51] And again a week later, when Hansen allows that it is especially grumbling people who get hit with the disease.[52]

In *Jørgen Stein*, Paludan mentions briefly that Jørgen is afraid when he visits Nanna on her deathbed, and there is a suggestion of an ethical dilemma when he has doubt over whether he should protect himself in a tense situation where he should be showing his love.[53] But the fear is described predominantly as an emotional tension in Jørgen's and Nanna's relationship, and the barrier raised by the disease as a tragic obstacle in an unhappy love story. Nanna slips back into memory and unearths all of the noncommittal approaches there have been between the two, and there is no room for general consideration of fear of contagion apart from their intimate relations. Here the novel distinguishes itself from Paludan's 1924 *En Vinter Lang* (A winter long), wherein the influenza epidemic also plays a role. For example, one hears how the news that the town's watchmaker's apprentice has died of influenza first leaves the townsfolk void of memory, but they slowly come to think of the way he would scrape the price sticker off of a watch with his fingernail and then spit-polish it.[54] It is a small obvservation, but with great meaning, as it portrays how the fear of contagion sneaks into daily life and memory.

At the same time, there are no descriptions in *En vinter lang* of the dilemma people found themselves in concerning the need to care for the sick. The low mortality meant that many lives could be saved if they only received the proper care, and there were many people who chose to defy the danger of contagion. Collier describes how a Danish nurse, Else Dahl, declined to honor her husband's prohibition against visiting the sick. He feared that she would being the disease home to the family, but she believed she was obliged to help and her Christian faith was a testimony to the great importance religion can have for the power of ethical engagements.[55] A similar story of a woman who came to the rescue of several families is told in Søren Skoubo's memoire.[56]

6. The Beautiful Corpse

Paludan describes the influenza as a horrible phenomenon that nonetheless has its own diabolical beauty. Its corrosion has transformed Nanna into a 'beautiful woman', and Jørgen is both attracted to and frightened by her roguish gaze, which seems alluring and coquettish.[57] Just in case the reader has not grasped the parallel between the prostitutes and the mortally ill Nanna, Paludan points explicitly to the blue-grey tone around her eyes and has Jørgen think about the loose women with shame and confusion. There are in this description, as in Thomas Mann, significant connections among sickness, health and nature. It was the 'childhood surplus', in which her parents are implicated, that made Nanna plump, while the disease has had the effect of 'regulating' her weight, making her so 'beautiful that it was painful'.[58] She lies in her sick bed, having difficulty breathing, gasping and coughing rather like a tubercular, but she remains composed and like Jørgen experiences their last meeting as a moment of truth. She makes it known that she has read Jørgen like an open book, and he conversely reveals his guilt, regret and repentance. It is an ideal death scene: beautiful, true and without too much pain.

In reality the course of the disease and deaths during the epidemic were less picturesque. This appears from Collier's and Barry's books, which are written in alternating styles, mixing technical and epical passages. Thus one finds graphic descriptions of how people attacked by viral pneumonia suddenly dropped dead in the middle of the street or on the train home due to liquid and debris-filled lungs. There are also accounts of nosebleeds, gangrene of the reproductive organs and all the types of pneumonia that could befall the influenza victims.[59] Furthermore, as Danish doctor Victor Scheel writes, the victims were often afflicted with psychic disorders and psychosis in the course of the disease.[60] Some deaths were quite different for Nanna's long illness and without her reconcilition with the past and immanent death. *En vinter lang* can also serve as an example of a different Paludanesque description of the death experience. In this case death is not described as a final stop after an intense crescendo, where the dying person achieves self-knowledge, but rather as the stopping point after a short interval of total alienation. Paludan first writes: 'One went to a ball on Sunday, and on Tuesday some strange, hard, unmoving and frightful plaster cast of oneself lay in one's bed, while relatives went about in whispers...'[61] Afterwards comes a portrait of Lassen, who is waiting to die and says darkly: 'Then a sentence comes, helter skelter – a dark universe of words, without a ray of reason'.[62]

In the first example from *En vinter lang* we also perceive a slipping away from the individual over to death as a common condition. It is 'one' who becomes infected and moves into death's realm. At the same time, the passae does not describe the horror of deatrh's unavoidable banality. If one further compares Paludan's novels to *Salige er de enfoldige* and *La Peste*, death in the latter pair is the turning point in a discussion between doctors and their opponents. Why fight against that which in any case comes upon us all unexpectedly one day? Why not give up, and let death take up even more space than it has already won? It is as if the disease has become a collective, anonymous entity, against which the many obituaries with individual names and ages are but a final and vain rebellion. In both Gunnarson's and Camus' novels one gains an insight into how it feels to be a nealy mechanical part of that entire apparatus that processes the sick and dying, from the ambulance service to the cemetary officials, with no end to the wretchedness in sight.[63] This portrait of death as a constant, calculated proximity is perhaps the more horrifying, and it is merely suggested in Paludan's novels.

In the essay 'Hospitalsfantasier' (hospital phantasies), which Paludan wrote in connection wiith an operation, one gets an impression of the foundation he could also have laid for his novel. The essay describes the hospital as an island in society, where the individual is confronted with the fear of disease and death together with the other patients, and where the health authorities' professional approach to death is frightening. He writes here that the solemn talk of disease does more harm than good. 'Rather the shining unsheathed scalpel than a cotton pack that bodes one's doom!'[64] And he tells how disagreeable it would be to die a 'good municipal will death' in the hospital ward.[65] Behind the whole piece is an uneasiness with death's banality and its reduction of the individual to part of the mass. But what is good for the doctor's tale is not good for the writer's, as the experience of sickness and death is not to be found in *Jørgen Stein*, despite their overwhelming proximity during the epidemic.

7. Conclusion

Jørgen Stein creates a strong inpression of historical actuality with its topographical description of Ålborg with its characteristic Budolfi Church tower along with the insertion of national events such as the Landsmandsbank's collapse and international events such as the First World

War. As is the case for many other novels, one must nonetheless about calling it on this basis an objective portrayal of a time and place. As literary theorist Frederik Tygstrup has pointed out, realism is a generally problematic designation, a cookie-cutter that imparts the same form to all works. The intention of the present article has been to break with the notion of the novel as a neutral contemporary portraiture and instead to consider it as a construction whereby various representations of the influenza can be staged. In Paludan's case, as said, it is my opinion that the epidemic is used as part of a theme of decay. Like Mann, Paludan portrays a respectable family, frightened and threatened, but still in Jørgen's case fascinated with external dangers. The small provincial town, Havnstrup, is shown as a secure resort town Jørgen has difficulty leaving, but also as a nook he must get away from in order to be challenged and tempted, first of all by the girls he meets. His love life is the novel's central source of suspense, and the fight between reason and uncontrolable fascination, between healthy living and the death instinct, are its poles. Topographically there is a tendency to see what comes from outside as attractive. The prostitutes and exotic girls, the coffee dealer's daughter Ellen and the foreign Lily electrify Jørgen in a whole different way than does Nanna, for whom he has a nearly fraternal love.

The influenza epidmic is in this representation a general threat of an unclear, mystical nature. Paludan in the crucial passage compares disease to a divine judgement, suggesting that Nanna might have psychic abilities than enable her to foresee her own death. At the same time, the influenza is set into a well known decadence topography, inasmuch as it focuses on southern Europe as a kind of crime scene, from which disease emanates, and by making the mysterious stranger into a salesman Paludan aims a critique at modernity and mobility. As mentioned, this could have been the basis of a broader sociocritical decadence tale, but the characteristic element of the influenza's portrayal is that it never attains the character of a wave in the novel. Its impact is limited to Nanna, and the depiction of her infection, sickness and death is more part of a love story with moral undertones than a description of society. There is a focus on Jørgen's fascination with sickness and death, and a connection is made between the death-marked prostitutes, the 'fallen' Nanna, syphilis and the Spanish Flu. More than dealing with a scientifically and ethically challenged world civilization, the novel deals with a little family threatened by various external evils that fits into a general figuration of destruction with historical roots.

Translation by Thomas Petruso

Notes

[1] See L Otto, 'Sygdommen kom som en Explosion'. Den spanske syge i Danmark, [''The disease came like an explosion'. The Spanish Flu in Denmark'], *Fortid og Nutid*, March 2003, p. 12.

[2] Around 1900 the death rate in Scandinavia was down to 12–14%. See M Vovelle, *La mort et l'occident. De 1300 à nos jours*, Gallimard, Paris, 1983, p. 507 and Mark Harrison, *Disease and the Modern World*, Polity Press, Cambridge, 2004, p. 142.

[3] See A W Crosby, *America's Forgotten Pandemic. The Influenza of 1918*, (1989), Cambridge University Press, New York, 2003, p. 115.

[4] T Kristensen, Jacob Paludans Roman' ['Jacob Paludan's novel'], *Politiken*, 10 March 1932, pp. 7-8; 6 September 1933, pp. 7-8.

[5] E Frandsen, *Aargangen, der maatte snuble i Starten* [The age group that had to stumble at the start], Gyldendal, København, 1943, p. 22. O Lundbo, *Jacob Paludan*, Hasselbalch, Copenhagen, 1943: p. 92.

[6] T Mann, *Der Zauberberg*, E. Fischer Verlag, 1924.

[7] Vovelle 1983, *La mort et l'occident. De 1300 à nos jours*, p. 652.

[8] A Camus, *Pesten*, (1947), Stjernebøgerne, København, 1958. The plague is not described, as commonly stated in literary interpretations of the novel, as an allegory for the German occupation.

[9] Paludan wrote about Mann's novels *Buddenbrooks* and *Der Zauberberg* in Thomas Mann, *Nationaltidende*, 5 October 1930.

[10] J Paludan, *Jørgen Stein,* Steen Hasselbalchs Forlag, Copenhagen, 1935, p. 12 (originally published in 1932 as *Torden i Syd* [Thunder in the South], and 1933 as *Under Regnbuen* [Under the Rainbow]).

[11] ibid., p. 32.

[12] ibid., p. 186.

[13] ibid., p. 34; 52.

[14] ibid., p. 399.

[15] ibid., p. 402.

[16] M Foucault, *Sécurité, territoire, population. Cours au Collège de France 1977–1978*. Hautes Études, Gallimard, Seuil, Paris, 2004. Paul Virilio, *Unknown quantity*, London/New York, Thames & Hudson/Fondation

Cartier pour l'art contemporain, 2003. See also Harrison, *Disease and the Modern World*, p. 145.

[17] A W Crosby, America's Forgotten Pandemic. The Influenza of 1918, p. xiii.

[18] Smittefaren paa Centralbanegaarden, *BT*, 11 November 1918. An analysis of a number of newspapers' coverage of the influenza pandemic is found in Lise Markussen, *'Den spanske syge' i Danmark*, Københavns Universitet, 2004.

[19] Den Spanske m.m., in *København*, 19 September 1918, p. 2.

[20] Den spanske Syge vedbliver at gribe om sig, in *Nationaltidende,* 20 October 1918, p. 5.

[21] Den spanske Syge, in *Nationaltidende,* 25 October 1918.

[22] Dagens Smil, in *B.T.*, 29 October 1918, p. 1.

[23] E V Jensen, *Journal* nr: 3118/1, Aalborg National Archives.

[24] M Åman. *Spanska sjukan. Den svenska epidemin 1918-1920 och des internationella bakgrund* (Spanish Flu. The Swedish epidemic 1918–1920 and its international background), Uppsala University Institute of History, Uppsala, 1990, p. 211. Crosby notes that in the United States one feared that the country's defenders, the soldiers, had suddenly become the greatest threat to the nation (p. 56).

[25] Fra Krigsskuepladserne, in *Socialdemokraten*, 30 June 1918, p. 1; København i Influenzaens Tegn, In *Socialdemokraten*, 22 July, p. 2. The article Den spanske syge, however, complains of the unsanitary conditions in the infirmary with a quotation from *Berlingske Tidende*, 15 August 1918, p. 5.

[26] Gaa ikke i Kirke i Morgen (Do not go to church tomorrow), In *Folkets Avis*, 2 November 1918, p. 3.

[27] See R Collier, *The Plague of the Spanish Lady. The Influenza Pandemic of 1918-1919*, London, Macmillan, 1974, p. 45 and J Barry, *The Great Influenza. The Epic Story of the Deadliest Plague in History*, Viking, New York, 2004, which elaborately analyses how American research initiatives were set back by the war.

[28] R Collier, *The Plague of the Spanish Lady. The Influenza Pandemic of 1918-1919*, p. 9.

[29] ibid., p. 82.

[30] ibid., p. 11.

[31] M Åman, *Spanska sjukan. Den svenska epidemin 1918-1920 och dens internationella bakgrund*, p. 210.

[32] Streptokokkernes fornægter (Streptococcus' deniers), in *Ekstrabladet*, 23 October 1918; Influenzaen, in *Socialdemokraten*, 11 July 1918, p. 2.

[33] The Spanish Lady has since become a cultural pet name as well as a dead metaphor. It can be compared to the Dutch Zwarte Piet figure, whose cruel story has been forgotten, according to Mieke Bal, 'Zwarte Piet's *Bal Masqué'*, In *Zwarte Piet, Anna Fox*, Black Dog Publishing, London, 1999.

[34] H Heidemann, 'Om 'den spanske syge' 1918-1920' ('On 'the Spanish Flu' 1918–1920'), *Medicinsk Forum*, 18(1), 1965, p. 16.

[35] Paludan, *Jørgen Stein,* p. 138.

[36] H Kurzke, *Thomas Mann. Epoche – Werk – Wirkung*, C.H. Beck, München, 1991, p. 200.

[37] Paludan, *Jørgen Stein*, p. 387.

[38] Collier, p. 40. Barry, 2004.

[39] Paludan, *Jørgen Stein*, p. 403.

[40] op. cit.

[41] O Thomsen, *Krigsepidemiologiske Erfaringer* (Experiences in wartime epidemiology), Militærlægeforeningen, København, 1919, p. 27.

[42] See E Tognotti, Scientific triumphalism and learning from facts, In *The Journal of the Society for the Social History of Medicine*, 16(1), 2003.

[43] As occurs in Lars von Trier's film *Epidemic*, 1988.

[44] G Gunnarson, *Salige er de enfoldige*, Gyldendalske Boghandel, Nordisk Forlag, Copenhagen, 1920.

[45] Crosby, p. 236.

[46] D Thomson and R Thomson, *Influenza,* Ballière, Tindall and Cox, London, 1934, p. 1243.

[47] O Thomsen, Nogle Leveregler i Anledning af 'den spanske Syge' (Some rules of conduct in connection with the Spanish Flu), *Berlingske Tidende*, 27 July 1918, p. 5.

[48] ibid.

[49] N K Bristow, You can't do anything for influenza: doctors, nurses and the power of gender during the influenza pandemic in the United States, and Wilfried Witte, The plague that was not allowed to happen: German medicine and the influenza epidemic of 1918-19 in Baden, In *The Spanish Influenza Pandemic of 1918-19: New Perspectives*, H Phillips and D Killingray (eds), Routledge, New York, 2003, p. 57. It could be articles such as these that provoked Roy Porter to argue for a more nuanced understanding of medical science than the discourse analysis critique of 'medical imperialistic suppression'. According to Porter, medical history was a bit too eager to jump on the discourse criticism bandwagon in the 1980s, when it replaced its traditional history's glorified description of doctors and medicine. Roy Porter, More than a Foreword, In *Cultural Approaches to the History of Medicine. Mediating Medicine in Early Modern and Modern Europe*, W de Blécourt and C Usbourne (eds), Palgrave Macmillan, New York, 2004, p. x.

[50] Omkring Bacillen, *København*, 21 July 1918, p. 3.

[51] Den Spanske m.m., *København*, 18 July 1918, p. 2.

[52] Fru Jensen m.m., *København* 25 July 1918, p. 2.

[53] Paludan, *Jørgen Stein*, p. 405.

[54] J Paludan, *En vinter lang*, (1924), Steen Hasselbalchs Forlag, Copenhagen, 1972, p. 46.

[55] Collier, pp. 46 & 117. See also Crosby, p. 115.

[56] Søren Skoubo, *Journal.nr. 906/1986*, Aalborg Stadsarkiv.

[57] J Paludan, *Jørgen Stein*, pp. 402-403.

[58] ibid., p. 404.

[59] Barry, p. 2; Collier, p. 38.

[60] V Scheel, Influenzaens klinik, In *Ugeskrift for Læger*, 81(15):p. 642.

[61] Paludan, *En vinter lang*, p. 47.

[62] ibid., p. 57.

[63] Camus, p. 135.

[64] J Paludan, Hospitalsfantasier, In *Aaret Rundt. Trykt og utrykt*, Steen Hasselbalchs Forlag, Copenhagen, 1929, p. 58.

[65] ibid., p. 60.

Bibliography

i. Books

Bal, M., 'Zwarte Piet's *Bal Masqué'*. *Zwarte Piet, Anna Fox*, London, Black Dog Publishing, 1999.

Barry, J., *The Great Influenza. The Epic Story of the Deadliest Plague in History*. Viking, New York, 2004.

Bristow, N.K., You can't do anything for influenza: doctors, nurses and the power of gender during the influenza pandemic in the United States; and Wilfried Witte, The plague that was not allowed to happen: German medicine and the influenza epidemic of 1918-19 in Baden. *The Spanish Influenza Pandemic of 1918-19: New Perspectives*, H Phillips and D Killingray (eds), Routledge, New York, 2003.

Camus, A., *Pesten*. Stjernebøgerne, Copenhagen, 1958, (1947).

Collier, R., *The Plague of the Spanish Lady. The Influenza Pandemic of 1918-1919*. Macmillan, London, 1974.

Crosby, A.W., *America's Forgotten Pandemic. The Influenza of 1918*. Cambridge University Press, New York, 2003, (1989).

Frandsen E., *Aargangen, der maatte snuble i Starten*. Gyldendal, Copenhagen, 1943.

Foucault, M., *Sécurité, territoire, population. Cours au Collège de France 1977–1978*. Hautes Étude, Gallimard, Seuil, Paris, 2004.

Gunnarson, G., *Salige er de enfoldige*. Gyldendalske Boghandel, Nordisk Forlag, Copenhagen, 1920.

Harrison, M., *Disease and the Modern World*. Polity Press, Cambridge, 2004.

Jensen, E.V., *Journal*. Nr: 3118/1, Aalborg National Archives.

Kristensen, T., 'Jacob Paludans Roman' *Politiken*, 10 March 1932; 6 September 1933.

Kurzke, H., *Thomas Mann. Epoche – Werk – Wirkung*. C.H. Beck, München, 1991.

Lundbo, O., *Jacob Paludan*. Hasselbalch, Copenhagen, 1943.

Mann, T., *Der Zauberberg*. E. Fischer Verlag, 1924.

Markussen, L., *'Den spanske syge' i Danmark*. Københavns Universitet, 2004.
Otto, L., ''Sygdommen kom som en Explosion'. Den spanske syge i Danmark' *Fortid og Nutid*, March 2003.
Paludan, J., *En vinter lang*. Steen Hasselbalchs Forlag, Copenhagen, 1972, (1924).
Paludan, J., *Jørgen Stein*. Steen Hasselbalchs Forlag, Copenhagen, 1935.
Paludan, J., 'Thomas Mann'. *Nationaltidende*, 5 October 1930.
Porter, R., 'More than a Foreword'. *Cultural Approaches to the History of Medicine. Mediating Medicine in Early Modern and Modern Europe*, W de Blécourt and C Usbourne (eds), Palgrave Macmillan, New York, 2004.
Scheel, V., 'Influenzaens klinik'. *Ugeskrift for Læger*, 81(15),
Skoubo, S., *Journal.nr. 906/1986*. Aalborg Stadsarkiv.
Thomsen, O., *Krigsepidemiologiske Erfaringer*. Militærlægeforeningen, Copenhagen, 1919.
Thomsen, O., 'Nogle Leveregler i Anledning af 'den spanske Syge'' [Some rules of conduct in connection with the Spanish Flu]. *Berlingske Tidende*, 27 July 1918.
Thomson, D., and Thomson, R., *Influenza*. Ballière, Tindall and Cox, London, 1934.
Tognotti, E ., 'Scientific triumphalism and learning from facts'. In *The Journal of the Society for the Social History of Medicine*, 16(1), 2003.
Trier, L. v., *Epidemic*.1988.
Virilio, P., *Unknown quantity*. London/New York, Thames & Hudson/Fondation Cartier pour l'art contemporain, 2003.
Vovelle, M., *La mort et l'occident. De 1300 à nos jours*. Gallimard, Paris, 1983.
Åman, M., *Spanska sjukan. Den svenska epidemin 1918-1920 och des internationella bakgrund*. Uppsala University Institute of History, Uppsala, 1990.

ii. Newspaper Articles

'Smittefaren paa Centralbanegaarden'. *BT*, 11 November 1918.
'Den Spanske m.m.'. *København*, 19 September 1918.
'Den spanske Syge vedbliver at gribe om sig'. *Nationaltidende,* 20 October 1918.
'Den spanske Syge'. *Nationaltidende,* 25 October 1918.
'Dagens Smil'. *B.T.*, 29 October 1918.
'Fra Krigsskuepladserne'. *Socialdemokraten*, 30 June 1918.

'København i Influenzaens Tegn'. *Socialdemokraten*, 22 July, 1918.
'Gaa ikke i Kirke i Morgen' ['Do not go to church tomorrow']. *Folkets Avis*, 2 November 1918.
'Streptokokkernes fornægter' ['Streptococcus' deniers']. *Ekstrabladet*, 23 October 1918; Influenzaen, in *Socialdemokraten*, 11 July 1918.
Heidemann, H., 'Om 'den spanske syge' 1918-1920' ['On 'the Spanish Flu' 1918–1920']. *Medicinsk Forum*, 18(1), 1965, p. 16.
'Omkring Bacillen'. *København*, 21 July 1918.
'Den Spanske m.m.'. *København*, 18 July 1918.
'Fru Jensen m.m.'. *København*, 25 July 1918.

Pathogenesis: Life, Literature and Animality Medical Theory and Biological Nihilism in Eighteenth-Century Thought

Johan Redin

Abstract
In the history and theory of vitalism there is an attraction to the idea the post-human. Throughout the eighteenth and nineteenth centuries there was a lively discussion about not only the origin and nature of mankind, but also of its future and progress. The belief in a biological teleology was seriously challenged by the temptations of a biological nihilism. The debate, that initially chiefly concerned materialists, opened up for radically new ideas on the concept of life and the evolution of Man. Turning to Friedrich Schiller, Karl Philipp Moritz and Honoré de Balzac, this essay explores the role of medical theory in the history of aesthetics and the traces of biological nihilism in literature and philosophy.

Key Words: Biology; eighteen-century philosophy; medical theory.

> Thus is man that great and true *amphibium*, whose nature is disposed to live, not onely like other creatures in diverse elements, but in divided and distinguished worlds.... In brief we are all monsters, that is, a composition of man and beast.
>
> Sir Thomas Browne, *Religio Medicic* (1635)

*****

1. Aesthetics: The Original Programme

That 'nobody as yet has determined the limits of the body's capabilities',[1] that we do not know what a body can do, was a significant question for Spinoza. 'For nobody as yet knows the structure of the body so accurately as to explain all its functions, not to mention that in the animal world we find much that surpasses human sagacity, and that sleepwalkers do many things in their sleep that they would not dare when awake – clear evidence that the body, solely from the laws of its own nature, can do many things at which its mind is amazed.'[2] In Spinoza's philosophy, body and mind are just two aspects of the same reality and both are subject to natural law: 'the first thing that constitutes the essence of the mind is nothing else but the idea of a body actually existing'.[3] Even if Man is totally subjected to *affects*, we find in Spinoza an utterly affirmative philosophy of the body. Spinoza did not care much for aesthetics; in fact there was no aesthetics at his time.[4] But what he called for, a philosophy of affects, is something that later would became a science of aesthetics.

Aesthetics, a word that exists in most of our western languages, has a quite peculiar history. Outside the academic discussion, aesthetics is associated with everything from cosmetics and management to sports and design. That it has something to do with beauty and art is often an immediate association though. Art and aesthetics is repeatedly understood as more or less synonymous subjects, although it is far from clear why this is the case. My current research and field of interest is the formation of the discipline of aesthetics in the eighteenth-century, and especially its relationship to anthropology, medicine and physiology (comparative anatomy).[5] In the perspective of our contemporary rather fuzzy concept of 'aesthetics', the relationship to medicine and biology seems far away. (Except for perhaps the association with cosmetic surgery.) The word that was introduced 1735 by Alexander Gottlieb Baumgarten comes from the Greek *aisthēsis*, which means 'perception' or 'to perceive' – that is: the perception of the external world by the senses.[6] The intention of aesthetics *as a science* was not primarily to found a theory of art; it should aim for 'the perfection of the sensitive knowledge as such' (*aestheticis finis est perfectio cognitionis sensitivae*).[7] This means that it first of all is the study of the senses – in its qualitative *as well as* physical conditions. In fact, as Baumgarten introduced this concept, the idea of sensations, perceptions and emotions was as much an epistemological problem (regarding logic and apperception) as a physiological one (that of neurology and theory of irritability).[8] Dieter Kliche has shown how close this conception of aesthetics was to the concept of *pathology*, and that is in its rhetorical tradition of *ethos* and *pathos* as well as the medical tradition of *pathologus practius*.[9] Since aesthetics is the study of sensuous experience as such, it is definitely a study of affects, passions and emotions (mental excitement: *Gemütsbewegungen*) in all circumstances possible. The word *passio* (*passion*) is the Latin translation of the Greek *pathos*, and *pathologia* is thus the discourse of passions – no longer in the Cartesian tradition of a passively subjected soul, but of an *actively* effective passion.[10] Particularly interesting is the different 'diseases of the soul' (*Krankheiten der Seele*) where psychosomatic drives causes disturbances in the emotional balance as well as disorders of imagination and perception. By studying the mental and physical reactions to strong emotions and affects, by entering the regions of the subconscious, aesthetics would become a technique of educating as well as suppressing the influence of the senses on the operations of the soul.[11] In cultivating the senses, Man is to become a *felix aestheticus*, an assumption that marks out the anthropological premise in Baumgarten's theory of aesthetics.[12]

What is evident in this conception of aesthetics is that it also represents a new conception of Man. In the philosophy of the eighteenth-century Europe there are at least two great divides that signify the beginning of a rethinking of Man. The first one is the well-known Cartesian distinction between mind and body into *res cogitans* and *res extensa*. The mechanist and iatromechanist perspective on machinic life was soon to be challenged by the vitalist perspective on life forces (notably in the works of George Stahl and Albrecht von Haller) and the struggle for a synthesis of mind and body (the unified law of *commercium mentis et corporis*). The second great divide is the post-rationalistic philosophy of Immanuel Kant and the rift between nature and freedom; or, restrictively between the *phenomenal* and the *noumenal* worlds of Man. Again, a similar struggle for a synthesis is evident in the philosophical as well as the artistic responses to Kant. The common notion in the juxtaposition of these two divides, is that aesthetics operated as a bridging or intermediate instrument in both occasions.[13] The union of mind and body was sought for in the faculty of the senses and the union of nature and freedom was sought for in the very possibility of self-reflection, will and subjectivity.

2. Medical Philosophy and/as Anthropology

With its groundbreaking synthesis of medical and philosophical theories, Ernst Platner's *Anthropology for medical doctors and philosophers* (1772) became an immediate sensation in the German philosophical debate.[14] Platner was a professor of both medicine and philosophy (including aesthetics) at the university of Leipzig, where he lectured on the idea of a science that would consider 'the whole of Man' (*der Ganze Mensch*).[15] The physical as well as metaphysical sides of Man has been investigated in several different disciplines, and he insisted that it is time to bring them all together into one science, namely anthropology. Platner's radical ideas was also influencing the arts: it triggered the idea of an 'anthropological' or 'psychological' novel in the works of Johann Karl Wezel, Karl Philipp Moritz, and Jean Paul Richter (who also was a student of Platner); and, not say the least, it was important for the *Sturm und Drang*-literature of Johann Wolfgang Goethe, Johann Michael Reinhold Lenz and Friedrich Schiller.[16] However, Platner was not the only one to insist on anthropology as a meta-science of Man. One of Kant's former students, Johann Gottfried Herder, goes even further in suggesting the abandonment of the traditional concept of philosophy in favour of a new science of Man: 'all of our philosophy has to become anthropology', since any 'philosophy must make the people to its centre'.[17]

The new perspective on Man as a psychodynamic being was made an important aspect where the mind (*Geist*) was understood as a superior mediating agent between body and soul. Hence, body and soul cannot be properly understood in their isolation, they simply have to be studied as a physical whole. Therefore, the 'separation' between 'the medical science [...] and philosophy' is a disadvantage for both since they have 'lost more than they had gained' from their differentiation.[18] As Platner's friend Michael Hissmann puts it: 'the philosopher must become a doctor and the doctor must become a philosopher'.[19] This view became characteristic for the new trend in the Enlightenment thought, the so-called 'philosophical doctor' (*philosophische Ärzte*), represented by physicians such as Adam Weikard, Marcus Herz, and Jacob Friedrich Abel.

The relevance of Baumgartens aesthetics is also made explicit in Platner's writings, though not without critique. 'The sensual (*Sinnlichkeit*) in the general and broad meaning of the word', Platner writes, 'is the blending of the spiritual and animal (*Geistigen und Thierischen*) in one living being'.[20] The many misunderstandings of the concept of 'aesthetic sensation' (*aesthetische Empfindung*) are because of Baumgarten's unlucky neologism; he had chosen to link his project to the Greek *aisthēsis* instead of the more accurate *pathos*.[21] What are to be investigated are *sensations* (feelings, sentiments, affects, passions) and their connections to the totality of life (that is both physical and spiritual life). Experience is a product of sensory organisation of inputs and information of the surrounding world, as well as an inner *Empfindung*, a feeling of one's self, existence and above all of *life*. Life in this sense puts the biology of its time on the edge. Does life, as a guiding principle or force in nature, has perception? Perception as a power within the power of life – in short: the life of life. When identifying the sensual as the blending of the spiritual and animal, Platner is also approaching what will be one of the most controversial questions of the eighteenth-century. In the words of Herder, the 'laws of human and animal nature' is 'the darkness in my labyrinth'.[22] This was a question that no philosopher or anthropologist could be indifferent to: 'It is simply madness [to think] that we are merely self-reflecting pure spirits, philosophical atoms in ourselves. [...] We are at once animal spirits (*Tierartiger Geister*)'.[23]

3. Animality and Individuality: The Tragedy of the Vast Mass of Humanity

Let us look at two examples from this period where the man/animal interconnection is elaborated. First we will turn to a medical treatise by the young Friedrich Schiller, who was trained as a doctor at the well-known *Karlsschule* in Stuttgart. Second, we will turn to Karl Philipp Moritz' *Anton Reiser* and the experience of becoming animal.

Schiller's dissertation *Essay on the Connection Between the Animal and Spiritual Nature of Man* (1780) not only challenged some of his teacher's conception of the mind/body dualism; it is also a highly non-conventional presentation of medical theories along with literary representations. What we today sometimes call 'medical humanities' is not a novelty of the late twentieth century. It is fully documented that, for instance, the physiologist and psychologist Jacob Friedrich Abel used literature, and above all Shakespeare, in order to teach the young medical students the psychological complexities of illness.[24] Apart from, in a strictly medical context, quoting Shakespeare, as well as his own (yet unpublished) play *The Robbers* (1781), there are also hidden quotes from Heinrich Wilhelm von Gerstenberg's tragedy *Ugolino*, a drama often regarded as one of the first dramas of the *Sturm und Drang*. In Gerstenberg's violent tragedy, the former ruler of Pisa is condemned to death by starvation with his family, and as a result of his stoic determination he resists the temptation of cannibalism and instead takes his own life. The struggle for survival, although not to the cost of the essence of humanity, 'teaches him that he is a luckless cross-bread of beast and angel'.[25] Instead of murder his family, *he survives – as a human – by taking his life*. (The paradox is also recognized in the enigmatic last lines in Schiller's text: '*death evolves from within life as if from its seed*'[26].) The ideal of stoic strength is used to show how the struggle between spiritual and animal nature in the end arrives at extreme situations – cannibalism, incest, atrocity, and murder – where the fundamental nature of humanity has to be defended from animal nature. Here, it is morality and above all the *power of will* that marks the greatest difference between man and animal, not rationality or even physiology. Hence morality is not given by itself in Man: it has to be fought for; it is born out of *conflicts* – internal as well as external.[27]

Although morality is the main purpose in most of Schiller's philosophical writings, especially in his essays on tragedy and aesthetics, it is not the centre of attention in his medical dissertations. The arguments are all based upon a set of psychophysical laws that should demonstrate how the mind is dependent of the body and the body is dependent of the mind.[28] Precisely as in his earlier, though rejected, dissertation on the *Philosophy of Physiology* (1779), Schiller tries to track down the 'intermediate force' (*Mittelkraft*) between mind and body.[29] This intermediate force is located in the nervous system, in Stahl's tradition designated as 'animal spirits', which according to Schiller are guided by the faculties of attention and instinct. In his *Essay on the Connection Between the Animal and Spiritual Nature of Man* the theory of intermediate forces follows this vitalist idea of nerve-spirits (*Nervengeisten*), but they are also expected in the relation between man and animal as such. The two dissertations consequently form a sort of chiasmic relationship between the four instances: mind and body, man and animal.

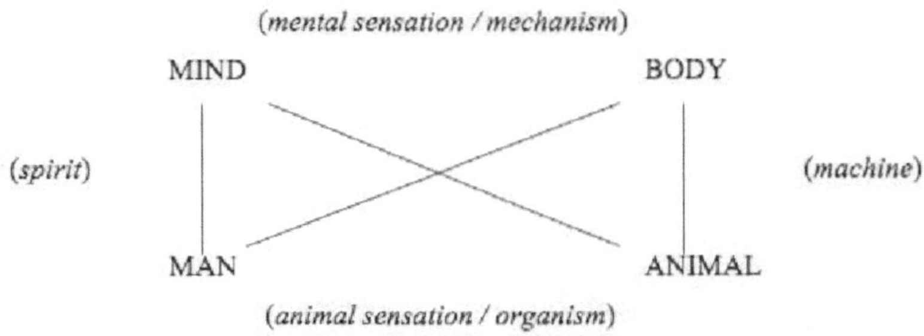

The bond between animal and spiritual nature is that of basic drives, needs and instincts on the one hand and the edifying, cultured and sensible on the other. Man is nothing but this essentially '*mixed* being' that cannot solely live in a world of abstraction and spirituality or totally run on her instincts and drives. The mind is taming the body (or rather 'shaping' it, as in Stahl's medical doctrine), and the body is refining the mind. Man 'had to be an animal before he knew that he was a spirit. […] *The body, therefore, is the first spur to action; the senses are the first rung on the ladder to perfection.*'[30] This is where Schiller's medical philosophy enter the original programme of aesthetics, including Platner's anthropological correction of Baumgarten's nomenclature: substituting *aisthēsis* for *patholgia*. Someone has to be in control of the 'machine', and the conflict between higher and lower levels of sensation remain absolute necessary in order to be a free, willing and thinking *subject*. Perhaps even more important is the dialectics of illness and health; Schiller would go as far as to say that illness and pain is required for keeping the animal and spiritual forces in conflict, and thus the 'most extreme bodily health hastens death as much as the most severe disease'.[31] Hidden as a minor footnote, Schiller also comes to something of a definition of the life of the animal. The 'animal life of the animal' (*tierisches Leben des Tiers*) depends on the 'experience of pleasant sensations', and it 'retains animal life' in that it 'lives today in order to survive tomorrow'. But this state of life is only an 'insecure state of happiness', because if the animal 'depends entirely on sensation' it is 'a slave to blind, random chance'. Schiller concludes:

> Man also live an animal life, experience pleasure and suffers pain. But why? He feels and suffers in order to preserve his animal life. He preserves his animal life in order to live a spiritual life all the longer. In this instance

> the means and the end differ; in the other end and means coincide. This is one of the crucial distinctions between man and animal.[32]

In contrast to Schiller's, we must say hopeful or at least balanced, analysis of man as this essential 'cross-bread of beast and angel', there is one remarkable depiction of the very breakdown of this balance. In Karl Philipp Moritz's 'psychological novel' *Anton Reiser* (published in three parts in 1785 to 90), we meet Man at the very fringe of animality; the becoming beast of humanity (with all the atrocities of the French revolution fresh in mind) and the becoming animal of intense sensations. Moritz, together with the philosopher Salomon Maimon, edited one of the first psychological journals, *Magazin zur Erfahrungsseelenkunde* (1783-92), where Platner's anthropology, together with an aesthetically oriented *Experimentalseelenlehre* merged into one powerful form of social psychology, a *Seelenkrankheitskunde*.[33]

In *Anton Reiser*, in many aspects Moritz's own autobiography, we follow Anton's struggle for respect and self-esteem through an almost constant humiliation from virtually every aspect of the *bürgerlische Leben* and social hierarchies. Precisely in the middle of the novel, accommodated on the loft of an old butcher's store, having witnessing the brutal execution of two criminals, Anton is close to a mental collapse. He is witnessing humanity itself at the guillotine. The vast mass of humanity is just a '*mass of human stuff*', in which everyone is a stranger and eventually '*lost amid the multitude*', so numerous that it at the same time is as 'insignificant' as 'the slaughter of an ox'.[34] Thinking about this humanity, 'that could be *cut to pieces* like an animal', made Anton 'compare himself to it mentally' and desperately searching for the essential 'difference between himself and such a slaughtered animal'.[35] Thus, he gradually begins 'to think himself into the being' of this animal. He wants to know the difference, so intensely that 'he would forget himself' and 'for a moment [believe that] he had apprehended the *nature of the existence* of such a being'.[36] Anton's intense feeling of becoming animal changes his existence, and Moritz is not hesitating in connecting Anton's becoming animal to the contemporary philosophical and medical discourse of the mind-body problem:

> he often wondered what it would be like for him if he were, for example, a dog living among people, or some other animal. – And as he had now begun thinking about the *difference between body and mind*, nothing seemed more important than to find, at the same time, some essential difference between himself and the animal, because he could not otherwise be convinced that the animal, whose

> body was so similar to his, did not have a mind like him. [...] These entirely sensual, animal ideas renewed his urge to live – he entirely forgot his humanity, just as he had done after the execution of the criminals, and returned home as an *animal* in his inclinations and sensations. As an *animal* he wished to go on living; as a human being, every moment his existence continued was intolerable.[37]

This '*being lost amid the multitude*', lost in the 'enormous mass of humanity [that] would turn into an equally enormous, shapeless mass of souls', brings Moritz' story an existentialist ground level of humanity. We remember Spinoza's saying that 'we do not yet know what a body can do', and this could as easily be added with the question if we yet know what the mind is capable of. What can Man become?

4. 'There is but one animal'

Throughout the eighteenth and nineteenth centuries there was a lively discussion about, not only the origin and nature of mankind, but also of its future and progress. The debate, that initially chiefly concerned materialists, opened up for radically new ideas on the concept of life and the evolution of Man. From Spinoza to Diderot, and from Schiller and Novalis to Balzac and Nietzsche, there are various philosophical as well as literary responses to this constructive materialism of potentiality. Nietzsche, who wrote 'for a species that does not yet exist'[38], made a 'humanity of the future' to a necessity in *Thus Spoke Zarathustra* (1883), with the so often misread slogan: 'Man is something that should be overcome'.[39] In the dialogue *d'Alembert's Dream* (written 1769, published posthumously 1789), perhaps the most radical view on life written in the eighteenth-century, Diderot suggests that the human being could just be any one of earths 'transient products,' because we 'now as little of what it has been as what it is going to be'.[40] The idea returns in Balzac's *Preface to the Human Comedy* (1842) as well, although in a different form. Those 'who insist on reading in me the intention to consider man as a finished creation', Balzac says, 'are strongly mistaken.'[41] It is noticeable that Nietzsche, as well as Diderot and Balzac, called attention to the relevance of medicine, physiology, and even zoology, in order to fully understand the *metaphysical* side of Man.[42] Balzac explicitly tells us that his idea of *The Human Comedy* first came to him 'as a dream', truly an 'impossible project' that 'originated in a comparison between Humanity and Animality'.[43] When contemplating the deeds of Leibniz, Buffon, Bonnet, Needham and Bichat, Balzac concludes:

> There is but one Animal. [...] 'The Animal' is elementary, and takes its external form, or, to be accurate, the differences in its form, from the environment in which it is obliged to develop. Zoological species are the result of these differences. [...] [But] does not society modify Man, according to the conditions in which he lives and acts, into men as manifold as the species in Zoology? [...] Thus social species have always existed, and will always exist, just as there are zoological species. [...] But the limits set by nature to the variations of animals have no existence in society. [...] [S]ome savants do not yet admit that animal nature flows into human nature through an immense tide of life.[44]

The last line is astonishing: neither science nor society is *yet* prepared to accept the animal nature that flows in our veins. Balzac's idea of sociology as zoology is to show metaphorically that 'there is no ontological break between the natural realm and the social realm'.[45] His enormous literary project thus coincides with biology in finding this *one and only animal* that is chosen to be an exemplar for a new species – the 'holotype'. Thus, as Allan Thiher emphasize, 'Balzac clearly believed that the ontology of fiction and of natural history coincide in this epistemological quest for the unique individual that is nonetheless the type for a species'.[46]

A closer look at the man/animal interconnections, way underneath the nebulous label of 'Enlightenment', reveals some quite astonishing ideas. In one of his final works, *The Conflict of the Faculties* (1798), Immanuel Kant challenges the widely held idea that 'the human species is constantly progressing to the better', by suggesting the possibility of a new revolution in the future of humanity. In his opposition to Peter Camper and Johann Friedrich Blumenbach, Kant's objection brings nature and politics in the closest contact possible:

> For, from the perspective of omnipotence of nature or, rather, from its supreme cause, which is inaccessible to us, the human being is only a trifle. But that the rulers of his own species also take him for one and treat him as such, partly burdening him as an animal, as a mere tool of their intentions, partly by exposing him in conflicts with one another to have him slaughtered – that is no trifle but an overturning of the *final end* of creation itself.[47]

In this passage, Kant is bringing two pieces together: the moral *ends* of humanity and Man as *means* of nature. Kant, if anyone, is known for his struggle for a strict boundary between man and animal, and even a distinction of man from every other form of organic life. As John Zammito says: 'the very idea of emergence or evolution in our sense *frightened* him'.[48] Nevertheless, the question that Kant actually proposes is: Since nature has its own chaotic way of reforming itself, then what if nature takes another route? Could there be another 'terrestrial revolution', as he is speculating in his *Anthropology from a Pragmatic Point of View* (1798), where 'the orangutan or the chimpanzee' could claim equal possession of the earth?[49] Peter Fenves has recently shown that the late Kant definitely was thinking of these possibilities, although it is in his marginal observations and footnotes.[50]

This thinking beyond Man is not exceptional for its age. The deeper the knowledge of the essence of life and matter, the more problematic it is to uphold the idea of anthropocentrism or anthropomorphic reasoning. In his penetrating study of the European Enlightenment, Panajotis Kondylis has effectively argued that the designation of this age is 'the ontological revaluation of matter' (*die ontologische Aufwertung der Materie*) and consequently two major tendencies that radically came to change both the natural and human sciences: the 'rehabilitation of sensibility' as well as the 'nihilistic distrust' (*Nihilismusverdacht*).[51] The reason for our existence suddenly turns out to be obscure, not to say accidental. 'Who knows', La Mettrie asks in his *Man the Machine* (1748), 'if the reason for Man's existence is not his existence itself? Perhaps he was thrown by chance somewhere on earth's surface, without knowing how and why – only that he must live and die'.[52] In Friedrich Schiller's tragedy *The Robbers* (1781), this doubt is echoed in the raging words of the materialist villain Franz Moor, who insists that: 'man originates from filth, wades for a while in filth, makes filth, and decomposes once into filth, until, in the end, he gets stuck as filth to the soles of his great-grandchild's shoes. That's the end of the song – the circle of human destiny in the muddle'.[53] From dust to dust, ashes to ashes, and from the ashes into the fire.

The idea of the teleology of Man was challenged by the temptations of a biological nihilism.[54] This somewhat dramatic concept was not used in the eighteenth-century (and perhaps it is not the best pick to use it at this point either). Biological nihilism should not be confused with mere misanthropy, or even atheism. What is meant is simply the distrust in the scientific explanation of rational causes, that our knowledge of nature could be nothing else than a fulfilment of the concept of reason that has been imposed on it. It is the very doubt of the idea of a given purpose in nature, where a moral or normative value has been ascribed to it. The writings of La Mettrie and above all marquis de Sade are clear evidence of this.[55] After the decline of physicotheology, the danger of relativism was always present in scientific explanation.[56] Nevertheless, the downfall of the idea of a presupposed natural order was not immediate; there was no sudden paradigmatic shift (Lamarckism did not end in 1859). This culminates in very the birth of biology as a concept, that is: *the abandonment of natural history (Naturgeschichte) for a science of life.*[57] The term 'biology' was coined in 1802 simultaneously and independently by Gottfried Reinhold Trevianus and Jean-Baptiste Pierre Antoine de Monet de Lamarck. The date is perhaps more than a symbolic coincidence: the turn of the century of Enlightenment as marking the move towards a 'positive science' based on the empirical knowledge of a unified programme.

5. Conclusion

Nowadays, when we talk about sciences as biology, psychology, or anthropology we have a quite clear conception of their disciplinary nature, although it is rather recently that these sciences has been differentiated from each other and institutionalised within different faculties. The perhaps most obvious divide is that between the human and natural sciences, between the study of Man as a physical being and a cultural being. In the late 1950's, C P Snow triggered the controversial debate about the 'two cultures' and their lack of communication and mutual ignorance of each other's practices.[58] This is a debate that still goes on, but I think that we still are far from the 'third culture' that once was suggested. In recent times the interactions between social science and cultural representation, law and literature, and 'medical humanities', just to name a few of the crossbreeds, are rather marginal projects. I think that a deeper interest in, for instance, the natural sciences and biology still is missing in the academic discussion of the humanities. The new and revolutionizing discoveries within genetics and biochemistry is about to totally reform our idea of life and technology, so it is surprising that this is met by silence in the humanities (although not in the arts). Once again the fundamental question of Man and above all the limits of the *concept* of Man is in the centre of attention; philosophical and ethical difficulties that should make a common ground for the natural, social and human sciences: What are we? Where are we going? What can we *become*? What I would like underline in this paper is that neither the notion of a 'third culture' or the idea of a transhuman being is a novelty of the twentieth century.

Since Foucault's biopolitical wake up call in the late 1970's,[59] the question of biopolitics has slowly turned into a new form of Life-philosophy, most recent in the works of Giorgio Agamben.[60] This is of course not the *Lebensphilosophie* of a Heinrich Rickert or a Wilhelm Dilthey; devoid of all Kantianism, it is a *political* interpretation of the *concept* of life. Although biology comes into question, it is not the biological conception of life that is important. It is an ethical life without morality, an organism without the organic, the life of the machine, the life of the apparatus of capture. It touches on the potentialities, capabilities and the boundaries of life. To reach to these boundaries one have to think beyond the human. As Deleuze and Guattari would have it: think of life's becoming *on the molar level*[61] – prior to the restrictions of life forms into different kingdoms of nature. Life is a kingdom without a king: it is a landscape of 'interkingdoms' (*inter-regnés*)[62] where monarchy has to become a polyarchy. This is no longer a Life considered by the natural sciences: 'Life alone creates such zones where living beings whirl around, and only art can reach and penetrate them in its enterprise of co-creation.'[63] As Diderot so beautifully put it: 'All nature is in a perpetual state of flux. Every animal is more or less a human being, every mineral more or less plant, every plant more or less animal.'[64]

Notes

[1] B de Spinoza, *Ethics*, in *Complete Works*, M L Morgan (ed), translated by S Shirley, Book III: prop. 2, Hackett Publishing Company, Indianapolis, 2002, p. 280.

[2] ibid.

[3] ibid., Book III: prop. 3, p. 282 .

[4] J C Morrison, 'Why Spinoza had no Aesthetics', in *Journal of Aesthetics and Art Criticism*, vol. 47, no. 4, 1989, pp. 359-365.

[5] This has recently been explored in the works of F Solms, *Disciplina Aesthetica: Zur Frühgeschichte der ästhetischen Theorie bei Baumgarten und Herder*, Klett-Cotta, Stuttgart, 1990; G Dürbeck, *Einbildungskraft und Aufklärung: Perspektiven der Philosophie, Anthropologie und Ästhetik um 1750*, Niemeyer, Tübingen, 1998; D Kliche, 'Ästhetische Pathologie: Ein Kapitel aus der Begriffsgeschichte der Ästehtik', in *Archiv für Begriffsgeschichte* 42, 2001, pp. 197-229; and H Adler, 'Aisthesis, steinernes Herz und geschmeidige Sinne: Zur Bedeutung der Ästhetik-Diskussion in der zweiten Hälfte des 18. Jahrhunderts', in *Der Ganze Mensch: Anthropologie und Literatur im 18. Jahrhundert*, H-J Schings (ed), Metzler, Stuttgart, 1994, pp. 96-111.

[6] Baumgarten's delineation of the concept of aesthetics is first and foremost in his major work *Aesthetica* (2 vol. 1750-1758), but Baumgarten's first use of the concept is in his dissertation on poetry: *Meditationes philosophicae de nonnullis ad poema pertinentibus* (1735), see the English

translation in *Reflections on Poetry: Alexander Gottlieb Baumgarten's Meditationes*, translated by K Aschenbrenner and W B Holther, University of California Press, Berkeley, 1954. A fully systematic investigation into the paragraphs of Baumgartens *Aesthetica* is offered in Michael Jäger's *Kommentierende Einführung in Baumgartens Aesthetica*, Georg Olms, Hildesheim, 1980.

[7] A G Baumgarten, *Theoretische Ästhetik*, H R Schweizer (ed), Felix Meiner, Hamburg, 1988, § 14.

[8] In this paper I leave out the important discussions in the French and British philosophical and psychological theory. For the discourse of the senses in the French enlightenment, see J C O'Neal, *The Authority of Experience: Sensationist Theory in the French Enlightenment*, The Pennsylvania State University Press, Pennsylvania, 1996. The British background with relation to European enlightenment thought is elaborated in the works of J W Yolton, *Perceptual Acquaintance From Descartes to Reid*, Blackwell, Oxford, 1984; and *Thinking Matter: Materialism in Eighteenth-Century Britain*, Blackwell, Oxford, 1984. Although O'Neal mentions Baumgarten, none of them links the British and French debate to Baumgartens aesthetical programme.

[9] Kliche (2001), 204 ff. My short hand presentation of the *aisthēsis – pathologia* problem draws heavily on Kliche's article.

[10] In the line of his aesthetic programme, Baumgarten will call pathology 'der Wissenschaft der sinnlichen Erkenntnis'. He also writes in his *Metaphysica* (1739): 'Da nun die Leidenschaften, einen starcken Einfluss auf die sinnliche Erkenntniss, und den Vortrag derselben, haben; so wird die Aesthetik auch, ihren Theil an der Lehre von dem Gemüthsbewegungen mit Recht fordern können' (quoted in Kliche (2001), 213). On Descartes' concept of 'passion', see Geneviève Rodis-Lewis's introduction, in R Descartes, *The Passions of the Soul*, translated and annotated by S Voss, Hackett Publishing Company, Indianapolis, 1989, xv-xxv.

[11] This is evident in the writings of the Baumgarten scholars Georg Friedrich Maier and Johann Christian Bolten. After reading Maier's *Anfangsgründe aller schönen Wissenschaften und Künste* (1750), Bolten suggests, in his *Gedanken von den psychologischen Curen* (1751), that 'die philosophische Pathologie ist die Lehre von denen Affecten, deren ästhetischer Theil lehret, wie man die Gemüthsbewegungen erregen, unterdrücken, und in seiner Gewalt haben soll' (quoted in Kliche (2001), 215). Aesthetics is

thus the science that gives the 'laws and rules' (*Gesetzze und Regeln*) for this technique, and Bolton gives plenty of suggestions: 'Die Aesthetick enthält die Regel der sinnlichen Erkenntniskräfte und des Vortrages derselben (§36); Die Aesthetick lehret ferner die Regeln, wie man die Sinne verbessern soll (§37); Die Aesthetick gibt uns auch die Anweisung, wie wir die Einbildungen erregen und unterdrucken sollen (§38); Die Aesthetick lehret die Regeln, wie man den Wiz verbessern soll (§39); Die Aesthetick lehret ferner, wie man die Scharfsinnigkeit verbessern soll (§40): Die Ae. lehret auch das Gedächtnis verbessern (§41); Die Ae. lehret, wie man die Dichtungskraft verbessern solle (§42); Die Ae. lehret, auch den Geschmack verbessern (§43); Die Ae. lehret, wie man Vorhersehungen und Vermuthungen hervorbringen und verhindern könne (§44); Die Ae. lehret endlich auch das Bezeichnungsvermögen zu verbessern (§45)' (ibid.). On Bolten, see also Dürbeck (1998), 132 ff.

[12] This has been emphasized by Steffen Gross, see 'The Neglected Programme of Aesthetics', in *British Journal of Aesthetics*, vol. 42, no. 4, 2002, pp. 403-414; and *Felix Aestheticus. Die Aesthetik als Lehre des Menschen*, Königshausen und Neumann, Würzburg, 2001. Cf. N Menzel, *Der anthropologische Charakter des Schönen bei Baumgarten*, Wanne-Eickel, München, 1969.

[13] See the second part in Dürbeck, 1998, pp. 115-316.

[14] E Platner, *Anthropologie für Ärzte und Weltweise*, Dyckische Buchhandlung, Leipzig, 1772. A revised second edition of this book appeared much later with a more accurate subtitle: *Neue Anthropologie für Aerzte und Weltweise. Mit besonderer Rücksicht auf Physiologie, Pathologie, Moralphilosophie und Aesthetik*, Crusius, Leipzig, 1790. Both editions state 'Vol. 1', but Platner did not continue any of the publications.

[15] See H-J Schings, *Melancholie und Aufklärung: Melancholiker und ihre Kritiker in Erfahrungsseelenkunde und Literatur des 18. Jahrhunderts*, Metzler, Stuttgart, 1977; H Adler, 'Aisthesis, steinernes Herz und geschmeidige Sinne', in Schings, 1994, pp. 96-103; and A Kosenina, *Ernst Platners Anthropologie und Philosophie: Der philosophische Arzt und seine Wirkung auf Johann Karl Wezel und Jean Paul*, Königshausen & Neumann, Würzburg, 1989, pp. 11-41.

[16] Although Platner was a prominent thinker of his time, it is only recently that his influence has been fully recognized. On Platner's influence on literary and aesthetic issues, see Schings, 1977; Kosenina, 1989; and C J.

Minter, *The Mind-Body Problem in German Literature 1770-1830: Wezel, Moritz, and Jean Paul*, Clarendon Press, Oxford, 2002.

[17] Herder, 'Wie die Philosophie zum Besten des Volks allgemeiner und nützlicher werden kann', quoted in Adler, 1994, p. 104.

[18] Platner, 1772, iii f.

[19] M Hissmann, *Psychologische Versuche, ein Beytrag zur esoterischen Logik*, Frankfurt und Leipzig, 1777, p. 22.

[20] Platner, 1790, p. 337.

[21] Platner writes in his *Anthropologie*: 'Der Ausdruck, ästhetische Empfindung, ist im Grunde freylich etwas sonderbar: de aber das Wort ästhetisch seit Baumgarten seine etymologische Bedeutung in dem Grade verloren hat, dass man kaum mehr daran denkt: so scheint es mir, wenigstens in systematischen Schriften, zur Bezeichnung der Empfindungen, die sich auf ästhetische Vollkommenheit beziehen, ein schickliches und fast unentbehrliches Beywort zu seyn' (Platner (1790), p. 337). This is even more emphasized in the § 92 of the second volume of his *Philosophische Aphorismen* (1782): 'Was wir in der Sprache der modernen Philosophie Empfindungen nennen, das heisst bei den Alten nicht aisthesis, sondern pathos, wie denn auch selbst Cartes und andere vor Leibnitzen das Wort passio noch in dieser weitern Bedeutung nehmen. Aisthesis heisst auch eigentlich nicht einmal die sinnliche Vorstellungen, sondern nur die körperliche Rührung der Organen.' What Platner had in mind was probably the stoic conception of *aisthēsis*, such as in the description in Diogenes: '*Aisthēsis* is the Stoics' name for the breath which extends from the commanding-faculty to the senses, and for the cognition of which they are instruments, and for their surrounding structure in respect of which some people get injured. The activity [of sensing] is also called *aesthesis*' (Diogenes Laertius, *Lives of eminent Philosophers*, Book VII, p. 52).

[22] Herder, quoted in John H. Zammito, *Kant, Herder, and the Birth of Anthropology*, The University of Chicago Press, Chicago, 2002, p. 333.

[23] Herder, quoted in Zammito, 2002, p. 317.

[24] On Abel's influence and psychological theories, see Kenneth Dewhurst and Nigel Reevs, *Friedrich Schiller: Medicine, Psychology, Literature. With the first English edition of his complete medical writings*, University of California Press, Berkeley, 1978, pp. 128-136; Wolfgang Riedel, *Die*

Anthropologie des jungen Schiller. Zur Ideengeschichte der medizinischen Schriften und der 'Philosophischen Briefe' (Würzburg: Königshausen und Neumann, 1989); and 'Influxus Physicus und Seelenstärke. Empirische Psychologie und moralische Erzählung in der deutschen Spätaufklärung und bei Jacob Friedrich Abel', in *Anthropologie und Literatur um 1800*, (ed.) Jürgen Barkhoff & Eda Sagarra (München: Iudicium, 1992), 24-52. Riedel has also edited a rich volume of Abel's documents: *Jacob Friedrich Abel. Eine Quellenedition zum Philosophieunterricht an der Stuttgarter Karlsschule (1773-1782). Mit Übersetzung, Einleitung, Kommentar und Bibliographie* (Würzburg: Königshausen und Neumann, 1997).

[25] Friedrich Schiller, *Essay on the Connection Between the Animal and the Spiritual Nature of Man*, in Dewhurst and Reevs (1978), 262. This quote is actually a paraphrase from Albrecht von Haller.

[26] ibid. 285.

[27] This is evident in Schiller's essays on tragedy in his journal *Neue Thalia* 1792, *Über den Grund des Vergnügens an tragischen Gegenständen* (first issue) and *Über die tragische Kunst* (second issue).

[28] There are two basic laws, see *Essay on the Connection…* § 12 and § 18.

[29] I have commented upon this thesis of Schiller elsewhere, see Johan Redin, 'Adventures in Bioaesthetics – Art, Biology and Aesthetic Experience in Early German Romanticism and the Art of Sturm und Drang', in *Nordic Journal of Aesthetics* 24 (2001), 131-149.

[30] Dewhurst and Reevs (1978), 270.

[31] ibid. (286).

[32] ibid. 260. Translation modified. Dewhurst and Reevs prefer in this context to translate *Tier* as 'Brute', which, I think, diminish the difficulty of the concept of animal in Schiller's text.

[33] On Moritz, see Schings, 1977; Raimund Bezold, *Popularphilosophie und Erfahrungsseelenkunde im Werk von Karl Philipp Moritz*, Königshausen und Neumann, Würzburg, 1984; M L Davies, 'Karl Philipp Moritz's Erfahrungsseelenkunde: Its Social and Intellectual Origins', in *Oxford German Studies*, 16, 1985, pp. 13-35; L Müller, *Die kranke Seele und das Licht der Erkenntnis: Karl Philipp Moritz' Anton Reiser*, Athenäum, Frankfurt am Main, 1987; and S Frickmann, ''Jeder Mensch nach dem ihm eignen Maaß': Karl Philipp Moritz' Konzept einer

'Seelenkrankheitskunde'', in *The German Quarterly*, Vol. 61, no. 3, 1988, pp. 387-402.

[34] K P Moritz, *Anton Reiser: A Psychological Novel*, translated and with an introduction by R Robertson, Penguin Books, Harmondsworth, 1997, p. 182 f.

[35] ibid., p. 183.

[36] ibid. Thus, it is not surprising that *the* philosophers of becoming, Gilles Deleuze and Felix Guattari, actually refer to this passage in *Anton Reiser*; see G Deleuze and F Guattari, *A Thousand Plateaus: Capitalism and Schizophrenia*, translated by B Massumi, Athlone Press, London, 1988, p. 240. Cf. also the reference in Gilles Deleuze's essay 'Literature and Life', in *Essays: Critical and Clinical*, translated by D W Smith and M A Greco, University of Minnesota Press, Minneapolis, 1997, p. 2.

[37] ibid., pp. 183-185.

[38] F Nietzsche, *The Will to Power*, translated by W Kaufmann and R J Hollingdale, Random House, New York, 1968, sec. 958.

[39] F Nietzsche, *Thus Spoke Zarathustra*, translated by R. J. Hollingdale, Penguin Books, Harmodsworth, 1969.

[40] D Diderot, *Rameau's Nephew and D'Alembert's Dream*, translated with introduction by L Tancock, Penguin Books, Harmodsworth, 1966, p. 154 (cf. 172 f.). On Diderot's transformist biophilosophy, see Lester C. Crocker, 'Diderot and Eighteenth Century French Transformism', in *Forerunners of Darwin: 1745-1859*, Bently Glass, Oswei Temkin and William L. Straus (eds), Johns Hopkins University Press, Baltimore, 1958, pp. 114-143.

[41] H de Balzac, *Introduction to the Human Comedy*.

[42] There is plenty of literature on this issue. On Balzac see for instance Graeme Tytler, *Physiognomy in the European Novel: Faces and Fortunes*, Princeton University Press, New Jersey, 1982; L Rothfield, *Vital Signs: Medical Realism in Nineteenth-Century Fiction*, Princeton University Press, Princeton, 1992, pp. 46-83; A Thiher, *Fiction Rivals Science: The French Novel from Balzac to Proust*, University of Missouri Press, Columbia, 2001, pp. 37-80. On Nietzsche see K A Pearson, *Viroid life: Perspectives on Nietzsche and the Transhuman Condition*, Routledge, London, 1997; and G Moore, *Nietzsche: Biology and Metaphor*, Cambridge University Press, Cambridge, 2002.

[43] H de Balzac, *Introduction to the Human Comedy*

[44] ibid.

[45] Thiher, 2001, p. 70.

[46] ibid.

[47] I Kant, *Streit der Fakultäten*, in *Werke in sechs Bänden*, W Weischedel (ed), Vol. VI, Wissenschaftliche Buchgesellschaft, Darmstadt, 1964, 362.

[48] Zammito, 2002, p. 306; cf. J H Zammito, *The Genesis of Kant's Critique of Judgment*, The University of Chicago Press, Chicago, 1992, 189-227. This is also brought up brilliantly in Susan Meld Shell's *The Embodiment of Reason: Kant on Spirit, Generation, and Community*, The University of Chicago Press, Chicago, 1996.

[49] I Kant, *Anthropologie in pragmatischer Hinsicht*, in *Werke in sechs Bänden*, W Weischedel (ed), Vol. VI, Wissenschaftliche Buchgesellschaft, Darmstadt, 1964, p. 682.

[50] P Fenves, *Late Kant: Towards Another Law of the Earth*, Routledge, London, 2003. In one of the notes in *Opus postumum* Kant states: 'human beings, as rational beings, exist for the sake of other human beings of a different species (races)'; the full passage runs: 'Man kann nun die Classification organischer und lebender Wesen noch weiter treiben da nämlich nicht blos das Gewächsreich um des Thierreichs und dessen Vermehrung und Vermannigfaltigung sondern Menschen als Vernünftige um anderer der Species (Race) nach verschiedenen Menschen willen da sind als welche um eine Stufe der Menschheit höher stehen entweder neben einander wie etwa Amerikaner und Europäer oder nach einander wenn durch Erdrevolutionen unser selbst organisirte vorher wiederum nach der Zerstörung ihrerseits anderen Platz machten und so die organische Natur in verschiedenen auf einander folgenden Weltepochen sich obzwar in verschiedenen Formen reproducirend und unseren Weltkörper nicht blos als ein mechanisch sondern auch organisch gebildeten Körper denken ließe. – Wie viel solcher Revolutionen unter denen zwar viele alte jetzt nicht mehr über der Erde lebende Organische Wesen vor der Existenz des Menschen vorher gegangen seyn mögen da jetzt kein einziges Exemplar (nach Camper) vom letzteren in den Tiefen derselben mehr angetroffen wird und welche vielleicht mit vollkommenerer Organisation noch bevorstehen dürften ist unseren ausspähenden Blicken verborgen.' I Kant, *Gesammelte Schriften*,

Akademie Ausgabe, Deutsche Akademie der Wissenschaften, vol. XXI, de Gruyter, Berlin, 1936, p. 214.

[51] P Kondylis, *Die Aufklärung im Rahmen des neuzeitlichen Rationalismus*, 2nd ed., Meiner, Hamburg, 2002, pp. 42 ff.

[52] La Mettrie, *L'homme machine: A Study in the Origins of an Idea*, A Vartanian (ed), Princeton University Press, Princeton, 1960, p. 176.

[53] F Schiller, *Schillers Werke*, Grossherzog Wilhelm Ernst Ausgabe, Max Hecker (ed), vol. 1, Insel Verlag, Leipzig, 1914. Cf. John Neubauer, 'The Freedom of the Machine: On Mechanism, Materialism, and the Young Schiller', in *Eighteenth-Century Studies*, vol. 15, No. 32, 1982, pp. 275-290.

[54] See S Moravia, 'From *Homme Machine* to *Homme Sensible*: Changing Eighteenth-Century Model's of Mans Image', in *Journal of the History of Ideas*, vol. 39, no 1, 1978, pp. 45-60; and Zammito, 2002.

[55] De Sade is brilliant in this, showing, on like two thousand pages of pornographic violence, that nature actually is to be regarded as a criminal according to the *scientific* norms of its actions!

[56] See W Lepenies, 'Naturgeschichte und Anthropologie im 18. Jahrhundert', in *Die Neubestimmungen des Menschen: Wandlungen des anthropologischen Konzepts im 18. Jahrhundert*, B Fabian, W Schmidt-Biggemann and R Vierhaus (eds), Kraus International, München, 1980, pp. 211-226. Important is also the chapter 'The Nihilist Dissolution' in Lester Crocker, *Nature and Culture: Ethical Thought in the French Enlightenment*, The Johns Hopkins Press, Baltimore, 1963, pp. 326-429. The first two chapters in Michael Allen Gillespie's *Nihilism Before Nietzsche*, The University of Chicago Press, Chicago, 1997 do also stress the origin in Descartes' methodological scepticism and mind-body distinction, although Gillespie's study do not have the scope we discuss here.

[57] The importance is stressed in Wolf Lepenie's influential study: *Das Ende der Naturgeschichte: Wandel kultureller Selbstverständlichkeiten in den Wissenschaften des 18. und 19. Jahrhunderts*, Suhrkamp, Frankfurt am Main, 1978.

[58] C P Snow, *The Two Cultures: and A Second Look*, Cambridge University Press, London, 1964.

[59] M Foucault, *History of Sexuality: An introduction*, translated by R Hurley, Random House, New York, 1978, pp. 133-159.

[60] See Giorgio Agamben, *Homo Sacer: Sovereign Power and Bare Life*, translated by D Heller-Roazen, Stanford University Press, Stanford, 1998; and *The Open: Man and Animal*, translated by K Attell, Stanford University Press, Stanford, 2004.

[61] G Deleuze and F Guattari, 1988, p. 275. Cf. the reconstruction of Deleuze's biophilosophy in Keith Ansell Pearson, *Germinal Life: The difference and Repetition of Deleuze*, Routledge, London, 1999.

[62] Deleuze and Guattari, 1988, p. 242.

[63] G Deleuze and F Guattari, *What is Philosophy?*, translated by H Tomlison and G Burchell, Columbia University Press, New York, 1994, p. 173.

[64] Diderot, 1966, p. 181.

Bibliography

Abel, J.F., Eine Quellenedition zum Philosophieunterricht an der Stuttgarter Karlsschule (1773-1782). Mit Übersetzung, Einleitung, Kommentar und Bibliographie. Königshausen und Neumann, Würzburg, 1997.

Adler, H., 'Aisthesis, steinernes Herz und geschmeidige Sinne: Zur Bedeutung der Ästhetik-Diskussion in der zweiten Hälfte des 18. Jahrhunderts'. Der Ganze Mensch: Anthropologie und Literatur im 18. Jahrhundert, Schings, H.-J. (ed), Metzler, Stuttgart, 1994.

Agamben, G., Homo Sacer: Sovereign Power and Bare Life. Translated by D. Heller-Roazen, Stanford University Press, Stanford, 1998.

Agamben, G., The Open: Man and Animal. Translated by K Attell, Stanford University Press, Stanford, 2004.

Baumgarten, A.G., Meditationes philosophicae de nonnullis ad poema pertinentibus (1735). English translation in Reflections on Poetry: Alexander Gottlieb Baumgarten's Meditationes, translated by Aschenbrenner, K. and Holther, W.B., University of California Press, Berkeley, 1954.

Baumgarten, A.G., Theoretische Ästhetik. Schweizer, H.R. (ed), Felix Meiner, Hamburg, 1988.

Bezold, R ., Popularphilosophie und Erfahrungsseelenkunde im Werk von Karl Philipp Moritz. Königshausen und Neumann, Würzburg, 1984.

Crocker, L.C., 'Diderot and Eighteenth Century French Transformism'.Forerunners of Darwin: 1745-1859, Glass, B., Temkin, O., and Straus, W.L. (eds), The Johns Hopkins University Press, Baltimore, 1958.

Crocker, L.C., Nature and Culture: Ethical Thought in the French Enlightenment. The Johns Hopkins Press, Baltimore, 1963.

Davies, M.L., 'Karl Philipp Moritz's Erfahrungsseelenkunde: Its Social and Intellectual Origins'. Oxford German Studies, 16, 1985.

Dewhurst, K. and Reevs, N., Friedrich Schiller: Medicine, Psychology, Literature. With the first English edition of his complete medical writings. University of California Press, Berkeley, 1978.

Deleuze, G. and Guattari, F., A Thousand Plateaus: Capitalism and Schizophrenia. Translated by Massumi, B., Athlone Press, London, 1988.

Deleuze, G. and Guattari, F., What is Philosophy?. Translated by Tomlison, H. and Burchell, G., Columbia University Press, New York, 1994.

Deleuze, G., 'Literature and Life'. Essays: Critical and Clinical, translated by Smith, D.W. and Greco, M.A., University of Minnesota Press, Minneapolis, 1997.

Diderot, D., Rameau's Nephew and D'Alembert's Dream. Translated with introduction by Tancock, L., Penguin Books, Harmodsworth, 1966.

Dürbeck, G., Einbildungskraft und Aufklärung: Perspektiven der Philosophie, Anthropologie und Ästhetik um 1750. Niemeyer, Tübingen, 1998.

Gillespie, M.A., Nihilism Before Nietzsche, The University of Chicago Press, Chicago, 1997.

Fenves, P., Late Kant: Towards Another Law of the Earth. Routledge, London, 2003. I Kant, Gesammelte Schriften. Akademie Ausgabe, Deutsche Akademie der Wissenschaften, vol. XXI, de Gruyter, Berlin, 1936.

Foucault, M., History of Sexuality: An introduction. Translated by Hurley, R., Random House, New York, 1978.

Frickmann, S., ''Jeder Mensch nach dem ihm eignen Maaß': Karl Philipp Moritz' Konzept einer 'Seelenkrankheitskunde''. The German Quarterly, Vol. 61, no. 3, 1988.

Gross, S., 'The Neglected Programme of Aesthetics'. British Journal of Aesthetics, vol. 42, no. 4, 2002.

Gross, S., Felix Aestheticus. Die Aesthetik als Lehre des Menschen. Königshausen und Neumann, Würzburg, 2001.

Hissmann, M., Psychologische Versuche, ein Beytrag zur esoterischen Logik. Frankfurt und Leipzig, 1777.

Jäger, M., Kommentierende Einführung in Baumgartens Aesthetica, Georg Olms, Hildesheim, 1980.

Kant, I., Werke in sechs Bänden. Weischedel, W. (ed), Wissenschaftliche Buchgesellschaft, Darmstadt, 1964.

Kliche, D., 'Ästhetische Pathologie: Ein Kapitel aus der Begriffsgeschichte der Ästhetik'. Archiv für Begriffsgeschichte 42, 2001.

Kosenina, A., Ernst Platners Anthropologie und Philosophie: Der philosophische Arzt und seine Wirkung auf Johann Karl Wezel und Jean Paul. Königshausen & Neumann, Würzburg, 1989.

Kondylis, P., Die Aufklärung im Rahmen des neuzeitlichen Rationalismus, 2nd ed., Meiner, Hamburg, 2002.

La Mettrie, L'homme machine: A Study in the Origins of an Idea. Vartanian, A. (ed), Princeton University Press, Princeton, 1960.

Lepenies, W., 'Naturgeschichte und Anthropologie im 18. Jahrhundert'. Die Neubestimmungen des Menschen: Wandlungen des anthropologischen Konzepts im 18. Jahrhundert, Fabian, B., Schmidt-Biggemann, W. and Vierhaus, R. (eds), Kraus International, München, 1980.

Lepenies, W., Das Ende der Naturgeschichte: Wandel kultureller Selbstverständlichkeiten in den Wissenschaften des 18. und 19. Jahrhunderts. Suhrkamp, Frankfurt am Main, 1978.

Menzel, N., Der anthropologische Charakter des Schönen bei Baumgarten. Wanne-Eickel, München, 1969.

Minter, C.J., The Mind-Body Problem in German Literature 1770-1830: Wezel, Moritz, and Jean Paul. Clarendon Press, Oxford, 2002.

Moore, G., Nietzsche: Biology and Metaphor. Cambridge University Press, Cambridge, 2002.

Moravia, S., 'From Homme Machine to Homme Sensible: Changing Eighteenth-Century Model's of Mans Image'. Journal of the History of Ideas, vol. 39, no 1, 1978.

Moritz, K.P., Anton Reiser: A Psychological Novel. Translated and with an introduction by Robertson, R., Penguin Books, Harmondsworth, 1997.

Morrison, J.C., 'Why Spinoza had no Aesthetics'. Journal of Aesthetics and Art Criticism, vol. 47, no. 4, 1989.

Müller, L., Die kranke Seele und das Licht der Erkenntnis: Karl Philipp Moritz' Anton Reiser. Athenäum, Frankfurt am Main, 1987.

O'Neal, J.C., The Authority of Experience: Sensationist Theory in the French Enlightenment. The Pennsylvania State University Press, Pennsylvania, 1996.

Neubauer, J., 'The Freedom of the Machine: On Mechanism, Materialism, and the Young Schiller'. Eighteenth-Century Studies, vol. 15, No. 32, 1982.

Nietzsche, F., Thus Spoke Zarathustra. Translated by Hollingdale, R.J., Penguin Books, Harmodsworth, 1969.

Nietzsche, F., The Will to Power. Translated by Kaufmann, W. and Hollingdale, R.J., Random House, New York, 1968.

Pearson, K.A., Viroid life: Perspectives on Nietzsche and the Transhuman Condition. Routledge, London, 1997.

Pearson, K.A., Germinal Life: The difference and Repetition of Deleuze. Routledge, London, 1999.

Platner, E., Anthropologie für Ärzte und Weltweise, Dyckische Buchhandlung, Leipzig, 1772.

Platner, E., Neue Anthropologie für Aerzte und Weltweise. Mit besonderer Rücksicht auf Physiologie, Pathologie, Moralphilosophie und Aesthetik, Crusius, Leipzig, 1790.

Redin, J., 'Adventures in Bioaesthetics – Art, Biology and Aesthetic Experience in Early German Romanticism and the Art of Sturm und Drang'. Nordic Journal of Aesthetics, 24, 2001.

Riedel, W., *Die Anthropologie des jungen Schiller. Zur Ideengeschichte der medizinischen Schriften und der 'Philosophischen Briefe'.* Königshausen und Neumann, Würzburg, 1989.

Riedel, W., 'Influxus Physicus und Seelenstärke. Empirische Psychologie und moralische Erzählung in der deutschen Spätaufklärung und bei Jacob Friedrich Abel'. Anthropologie und Literatur um 1800, Barkhoff, J. and Sagarra, E. (eds), Iudicium, München, 1992.

Rodis-Lewis, G., 'Introduction'. R Descartes, The Passions of the Soul. Translated and annotated by Voss, S., Hackett Publishing Company, Indianapolis, 1989.

Schings, H.-J., Melancholie und Aufklärung: Melancholiker und ihre Kritiker in Erfahrungsseelenkunde und Literatur des 18. Jahrhunderts. Metzler, Stuttgart, 1977.

Rothfield, L., Vital Signs: Medical Realism in Nineteenth-Century Fiction. Princeton University Press, Princeton, 1992.

Schiller, F., Schillers Werke, Grossherzog Wilhelm Ernst Ausgabe, Hecker, M. (ed), Insel Verlag, Leipzig, 1914.

Shell, S.M., The Embodiment of Reason: Kant on Spirit, Generation, and Community. The University of Chicago Press, Chicago, 1996.

Snow, C.P., The Two Cultures: and A Second Look. Cambridge University Press, London, 1964.

Solms, F., Disciplina Aesthetica: Zur Frühgeschichte der ästhetischen Theorie bei Baumgarten und Herder. Klett-Cotta, Stuttgart, 1990.

Spinoza, B. de, Ethics. In Complete Works, Morgan, M.L. (ed), translated by Shirley, S., Hackett Publishing Company, Indianapolis, 2002.

Thiher, A., Fiction Rivals Science: The French Novel from Balzac to Proust. University of Missouri Press, Columbia, 2001.

Tytler, G., Physiognomy in the European Novel: Faces and Fortunes. Princeton University Press, New Jersey, 1982.

Yolton, J.W., Perceptual Acquaintance From Descartes to Reid. Blackwell, Oxford, 1984.

Yolton, J.W., Thinking Matter: Materialism in Eighteenth-Century Britain. Blackwell, Oxford, 1984.

Zammito, J.H., The Genesis of Kant's Critique of Judgment. The University of Chicago Press, Chicago, 1992.

Zammito, J.H., Kant, Herder, and the Birth of Anthropology. The University of Chicago Press, Chicago, 2002.

Note on the Contributors

Hilde Bondevik, Ph.D., is associate professor at Centre for Gender Research, University of Oslo, Norway.

Hélène Cixous is writer, playwright, philosopher, literary critic and professor at University of Paris VIII, Paris, France.

Vincent Colapietro is professor of philosophy at the Pennsylvania State University, Pennsylvania, USA.

Gérard Danou, MD, Dr. ès lettres, works as physician in a hospital near Paris and as professor at Universities of Paris VII Denis Diderot and Cergy Pontoise, France.

Drude von der Fehr, Dr.art., is professor of comparative literature at the University of Oslo, Norway.

Jan C. Frich, MD, Dr.med., is neurologist at Department of Neurology, Rikshospitalet University Hospital, Oslo, and researcher at the University of Oslo, Norway.

Eric Hamraouï is Docteur en philosophie, maître de conférences and researcher at Conservatoire National des Arts et Métiers, Paris, France.

Deborah Kirklin is MD, Honorary Senior Lecturer in Medical Ethics and Humanities, University College London, UK.

Anne Kveim Lie, MD, Dr.med., is associate professor at Institute of General Practice and Community Medicine, University of Oslo, Norway.

Mette Kia Krabbe Meyer, Ph.D., is curator at The Steno Museum, Aarhus, Denmark.

Johan Redin, Ph.D., is associate professor at Uppsala University, Sweden.

Knut Stene-Johansen, Dr.philos., is professor of comparative literature at the University of Oslo, Norway.

Frederik Tygstrup is academic director of the Copenhagen Doctoral School in Cultural Studies, University of Copenhagen, Denmark.

www.ingramcontent.com/pod-product-compliance
Lightning Source LLC
Chambersburg PA
CBHW031322230926
51848CB00001B/59
9789042029439